Mometrix
TEST PREPARATION

CRES

Exam Secrets Study Guide

Dear Future Exam Success Story

First of all, **THANK YOU** for purchasing Mometrix study materials!

Second, congratulations! You are one of the few determined test-takers who are committed to doing whatever it takes to excel on your exam. **You have come to the right place.** We developed these study materials with one goal in mind: to deliver you the information you need in a format that's concise and easy to use.

In addition to optimizing your guide for the content of the test, we've outlined our recommended steps for breaking down the preparation process into small, attainable goals so you can make sure you stay on track.

We've also analyzed the entire test-taking process, identifying the most common pitfalls and showing how you can overcome them and be ready for any curveball the test throws you.

Standardized testing is one of the biggest obstacles on your road to success, which only increases the importance of doing well in the high-pressure, high-stakes environment of test day. Your results on this test could have a significant impact on your future, and this guide provides the information and practical advice to help you achieve your full potential on test day.

Your success is our success

We would love to hear from you! If you would like to share the story of your exam success or if you have any questions or comments in regard to our products, please contact us at **800-673-8175** or **support@mometrix.com**.

Thanks again for your business and we wish you continued success!

Sincerely,
The Mometrix Test Preparation Team

Need more help? Check out our flashcards at:
http://MometrixFlashcards.com/CRES

Written and edited by the Mometrix Exam Secrets Test Prep Team
Printed in the United States of America

Table of Contents

Introduction

Thank you for purchasing this resource! You have made the choice to prepare yourself for a test that could have a huge impact on your future, and this guide is designed to help you be fully ready for test day. Obviously, it's important to have a solid understanding of the test material, but you also need to be prepared for the unique environment and stressors of the test, so that you can perform to the best of your abilities.

For this purpose, the first section that appears in this guide is the **Secret Keys**. We've devoted countless hours to meticulously researching what works and what doesn't, and we've boiled down our findings to the five most impactful steps you can take to improve your performance on the test. We start at the beginning with study planning and move through the preparation process, all the way to the testing strategies that will help you get the most out of what you know when you're finally sitting in front of the test.

We recommend that you start preparing for your test as far in advance as possible. However, if you've bought this guide as a last-minute study resource and only have a few days before your test, we recommend that you skip over the first two Secret Keys since they address a long-term study plan.

If you struggle with **test anxiety**, we strongly encourage you to check out our recommendations for how you can overcome it. Test anxiety is a formidable foe, but it can be beaten, and we want to make sure you have the tools you need to defeat it.

Secret Key 1: Plan Big, Study Small

There's a lot riding on your performance. If you want to ace this test, you're going to need to keep your skills sharp and the material fresh in your mind. You need a plan that lets you review everything you need to know while still fitting in your schedule. We'll break this strategy down into three categories.

Information Organization

Start with the information you already have: the official test outline. From this, you can make a complete list of all the concepts you need to cover before the test. Organize these concepts into groups that can be studied together, and create a list of any related vocabulary you need to learn so you can brush up on any difficult terms. You'll want to keep this vocabulary list handy once you actually start studying since you may need to add to it along the way.

Time Management

Once you have your set of study concepts, decide how to spread them out over the time you have left before the test. Break your study plan into small, clear goals so you have a manageable task for each day and know exactly what you're doing. Then just focus on one small step at a time. When you manage your time this way, you don't need to spend hours at a time studying. Studying a small block of content for a short period each day helps you retain information better and avoid stressing over how much you have left to do. You can relax knowing that you have a plan to cover everything in time. In order for this strategy to be effective though, you have to start studying early and stick to your schedule. Avoid the exhaustion and futility that comes from last-minute cramming!

Study Environment

The environment you study in has a big impact on your learning. Studying in a coffee shop, while probably more enjoyable, is not likely to be as fruitful as studying in a quiet room. It's important to keep distractions to a minimum. You're only planning to study for a short block of time, so make the most of it. Don't pause to check your phone or get up to find a snack. It's also important to **avoid multitasking**. Research has consistently shown that multitasking will make your studying dramatically less effective. Your study area should also be comfortable and well-lit so you don't have the distraction of straining your eyes or sitting on an uncomfortable chair.

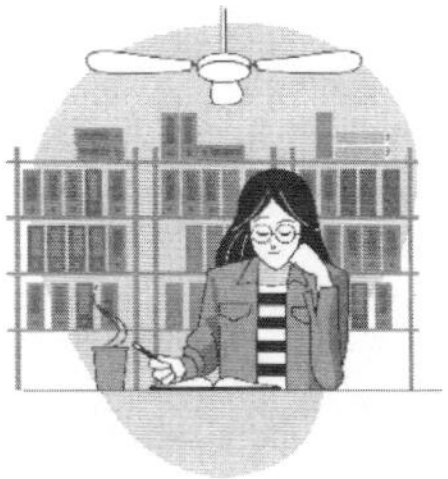

The time of day you study is also important. You want to be rested and alert. Don't wait until just before bedtime. Study when you'll be most likely to comprehend and remember. Even better, if you know what time of day your test will be, set that time aside for study. That way your brain will be used to working on that subject at that specific time and you'll have a better chance of recalling information.

Finally, it can be helpful to team up with others who are studying for the same test. Your actual studying should be done in as isolated an environment as possible, but the work of organizing the information and setting up the study plan can be divided up. In between study sessions, you can discuss with your teammates the concepts that you're all studying and quiz each other on the details. Just be sure that your teammates are as serious about the test as you are. If you find that your study time is being replaced with social time, you might need to find a new team.

Secret Key 2: Make Your Studying Count

You're devoting a lot of time and effort to preparing for this test, so you want to be absolutely certain it will pay off. This means doing more than just reading the content and hoping you can remember it on test day. It's important to make every minute of study count. There are two main areas you can focus on to make your studying count.

Retention

It doesn't matter how much time you study if you can't remember the material. You need to make sure you are retaining the concepts. To check your retention of the information you're learning, try recalling it at later times with minimal prompting. Try carrying around flashcards and glance at one or two from time to time or ask a friend who's also studying for the test to quiz you.

To enhance your retention, look for ways to put the information into practice so that you can apply it rather than simply recalling it. If you're using the information in practical ways, it will be much easier to remember. Similarly, it helps to solidify a concept in your mind if you're not only reading it to yourself but also explaining it to someone else. Ask a friend to let you teach them about a concept you're a little shaky on (or speak aloud to an imaginary audience if necessary). As you try to summarize, define, give examples, and answer your friend's questions, you'll understand the concepts better and they will stay with you longer. Finally, step back for a big picture view and ask yourself how each piece of information fits with the whole subject. When you link the different concepts together and see them working together as a whole, it's easier to remember the individual components.

Finally, practice showing your work on any multi-step problems, even if you're just studying. Writing out each step you take to solve a problem will help solidify the process in your mind, and you'll be more likely to remember it during the test.

Modality

Modality simply refers to the means or method by which you study. Choosing a study modality that fits your own individual learning style is crucial. No two people learn best in exactly the same way, so it's important to know your strengths and use them to your advantage.

For example, if you learn best by visualization, focus on visualizing a concept in your mind and draw an image or a diagram. Try color-coding your notes, illustrating them, or creating symbols that will trigger your mind to recall a learned concept. If you learn best by hearing or discussing information, find a study partner who learns the same way or read aloud to yourself. Think about how to put the information in your own words. Imagine that you are giving a lecture on the topic and record yourself so you can listen to it later.

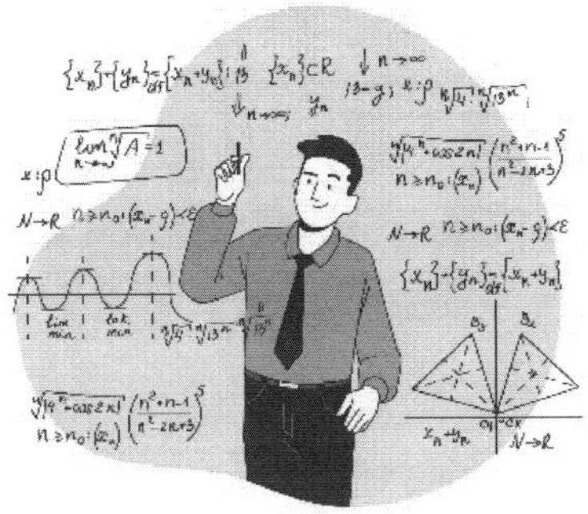

For any learning style, flashcards can be helpful. Organize the information so you can take advantage of spare moments to review. Underline key words or phrases. Use different colors for different categories. Mnemonic devices (such as creating a short list in which every item starts with the same letter) can also help with retention. Find what works best for you and use it to store the information in your mind most effectively and easily.

Secret Key 3: Practice the Right Way

Your success on test day depends not only on how many hours you put into preparing, but also on whether you prepared the right way. It's good to check along the way to see if your studying is paying off. One of the most effective ways to do this is by taking practice tests to evaluate your progress. Practice tests are useful because they show exactly where you need to improve. Every time you take a practice test, pay special attention to these three groups of questions:

- The questions you got wrong
- The questions you had to guess on, even if you guessed right
- The questions you found difficult or slow to work through

This will show you exactly what your weak areas are, and where you need to devote more study time. Ask yourself why each of these questions gave you trouble. Was it because you didn't understand the material? Was it because you didn't remember the vocabulary? Do you need more repetitions on this type of question to build speed and confidence? Dig into those questions and figure out how you can strengthen your weak areas as you go back to review the material.

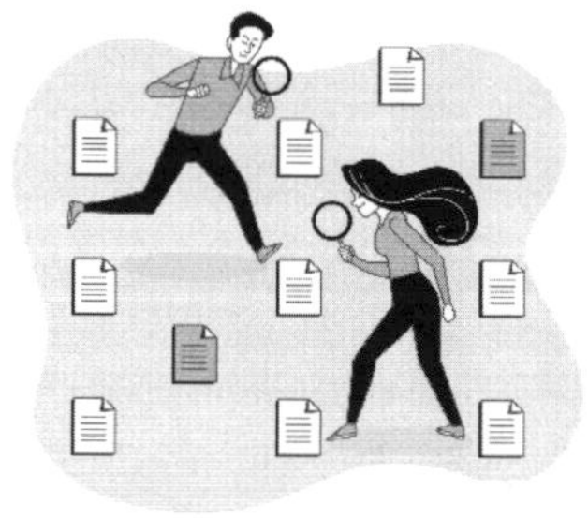

Additionally, many practice tests have a section explaining the answer choices. It can be tempting to read the explanation and think that you now have a good understanding of the concept. However, an explanation likely only covers part of the question's broader context. Even if the explanation makes perfect sense, **go back and investigate** every concept related to the question until you're positive you have a thorough understanding.

As you go along, keep in mind that the practice test is just that: practice. Memorizing these questions and answers will not be very helpful on the actual test because it is unlikely to have any of the same exact questions. If you only know the right answers to the sample questions, you won't be prepared for the real thing. **Study the concepts** until you understand them fully, and then you'll be able to answer any question that shows up on the test.

It's important to wait on the practice tests until you're ready. If you take a test on your first day of study, you may be overwhelmed by the amount of material covered and how much you need to learn. Work up to it gradually.

On test day, you'll need to be prepared for answering questions, managing your time, and using the test-taking strategies you've learned. It's a lot to balance, like a mental marathon that will have a big impact on your future. Like training for a marathon, you'll need to start slowly and work your way up. When test day arrives, you'll be ready.

Start with the strategies you've read in the first two Secret Keys—plan your course and study in the way that works best for you. If you have time, consider using multiple study resources to get different approaches to the same concepts. It can be helpful to see difficult concepts from more than one angle. Then find a good source for practice tests. Many times, the test website will suggest potential study resources or provide sample tests.

Practice Test Strategy

If you're able to find at least three practice tests, we recommend this strategy:

Untimed and Open-Book Practice

Take the first test with no time constraints and with your notes and study guide handy. Take your time and focus on applying the strategies you've learned.

Timed and Open-Book Practice

Take the second practice test open-book as well, but set a timer and practice pacing yourself to finish in time.

Timed and Closed-Book Practice

Take any other practice tests as if it were test day. Set a timer and put away your study materials. Sit at a table or desk in a quiet room, imagine yourself at the testing center, and answer questions as quickly and accurately as possible.

Keep repeating timed and closed-book tests on a regular basis until you run out of practice tests or it's time for the actual test. Your mind will be ready for the schedule and stress of test day, and you'll be able to focus on recalling the material you've learned.

Secret Key 4: Pace Yourself

Once you're fully prepared for the material on the test, your biggest challenge on test day will be managing your time. Just knowing that the clock is ticking can make you panic even if you have plenty of time left. Work on pacing yourself so you can build confidence against the time constraints of the exam. Pacing is a difficult skill to master, especially in a high-pressure environment, so **practice is vital**.

Set time expectations for your pace based on how much time is available. For example, if a section has 60 questions and the time limit is 30 minutes, you know you have to average 30 seconds or less per question in order to answer them all. Although 30 seconds is the hard limit, set 25 seconds per question as your goal, so you reserve extra time to spend on harder questions. When you budget extra time for the harder questions, you no longer have any reason to stress when those questions take longer to answer.

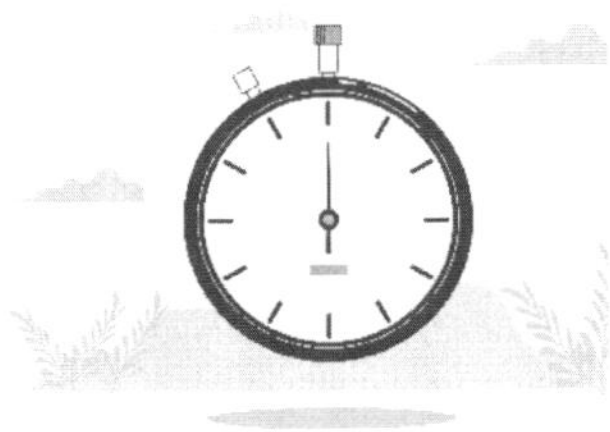

Don't let this time expectation distract you from working through the test at a calm, steady pace, but keep it in mind so you don't spend too much time on any one question. Recognize that taking extra time on one question you don't understand may keep you from answering two that you do understand later in the test. If your time limit for a question is up and you're still not sure of the answer, mark it and move on, and come back to it later if the time and the test format allow. If the testing format doesn't allow you to return to earlier questions, just make an educated guess; then put it out of your mind and move on.

On the easier questions, be careful not to rush. It may seem wise to hurry through them so you have more time for the challenging ones, but it's not worth missing one if you know the concept and just didn't take the time to read the question fully. Work efficiently but make sure you understand the question and have looked at all of the answer choices, since more than one may seem right at first.

Even if you're paying attention to the time, you may find yourself a little behind at some point. You should speed up to get back on track, but do so wisely. Don't panic; just take a few seconds less on each question until you're caught up. Don't guess without thinking, but do look through the answer choices and eliminate any you know are wrong. If you can get down to two choices, it is often worthwhile to guess from those. Once you've chosen an answer, move on and don't dwell on any that you skipped or had to hurry through. If a question was taking too long, chances are it was one of the harder ones, so you weren't as likely to get it right anyway.

On the other hand, if you find yourself getting ahead of schedule, it may be beneficial to slow down a little. The more quickly you work, the more likely you are to make a careless mistake that will affect your score. You've budgeted time for each question, so don't be afraid to spend that time. Practice an efficient but careful pace to get the most out of the time you have.

Secret Key 5: Have a Plan for Guessing

When you're taking the test, you may find yourself stuck on a question. Some of the answer choices seem better than others, but you don't see the one answer choice that is obviously correct. What do you do?

The scenario described above is very common, yet most test takers have not effectively prepared for it. Developing and practicing a plan for guessing may be one of the single most effective uses of your time as you get ready for the exam.

In developing your plan for guessing, there are three questions to address:

- When should you start the guessing process?
- How should you narrow down the choices?
- Which answer should you choose?

When to Start the Guessing Process

Unless your plan for guessing is to select C every time (which, despite its merits, is not what we recommend), you need to leave yourself enough time to apply your answer elimination strategies. Since you have a limited amount of time for each question, that means that if you're going to give yourself the best shot at guessing correctly, you have to decide quickly whether or not you will guess.

Of course, the best-case scenario is that you don't have to guess at all, so first, see if you can answer the question based on your knowledge of the subject and basic reasoning skills. Focus on the key words in the question and try to jog your memory of related topics. Give yourself a chance to bring the knowledge to mind, but once you realize that you don't have (or you can't access) the knowledge you need to answer the question, it's time to start the guessing process.

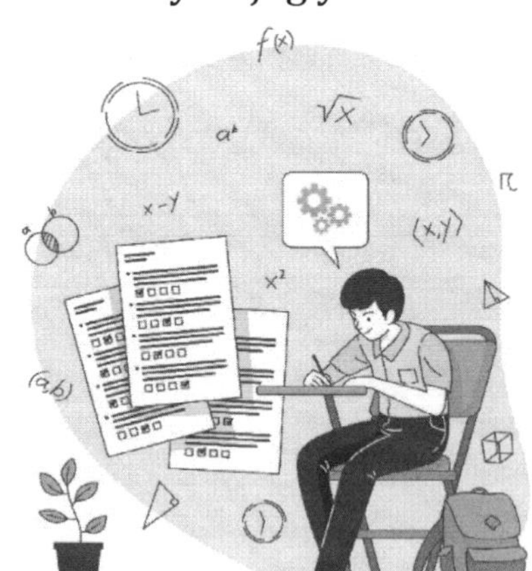

It's almost always better to start the guessing process too early than too late. It only takes a few seconds to remember something and answer the question from knowledge. Carefully eliminating wrong answer choices takes longer. Plus, going through the process of eliminating answer choices can actually help jog your memory.

Summary: Start the guessing process as soon as you decide that you can't answer the question based on your knowledge.

How to Narrow Down the Choices

The next chapter in this book (**Test-Taking Strategies**) includes a wide range of strategies for how to approach questions and how to look for answer choices to eliminate. You will definitely want to read those carefully, practice them, and figure out which ones work best for you. Here though, we're going to address a mindset rather than a particular strategy.

Your odds of guessing an answer correctly depend on how many options you are choosing from.

Number of options left	5	4	3	2	1
Odds of guessing correctly	20%	25%	33%	50%	100%

You can see from this chart just how valuable it is to be able to eliminate incorrect answers and make an educated guess, but there are two things that many test takers do that cause them to miss out on the benefits of guessing:

- Accidentally eliminating the correct answer
- Selecting an answer based on an impression

We'll look at the first one here, and the second one in the next section.

To avoid accidentally eliminating the correct answer, we recommend a thought exercise called **the $5 challenge**. In this challenge, you only eliminate an answer choice from contention if you are willing to bet $5 on it being wrong. Why $5? Five dollars is a small but not insignificant amount of money. It's an amount you could afford to lose but wouldn't want to throw away. And while losing $5 once might not hurt too much, doing it twenty times will set you back $100. In the same way, each small decision you make—eliminating a choice here, guessing on a question there—won't by itself impact your score very much, but when you put them all together, they can make a big difference. By holding each answer choice elimination decision to a higher standard, you can reduce the risk of accidentally eliminating the correct answer.

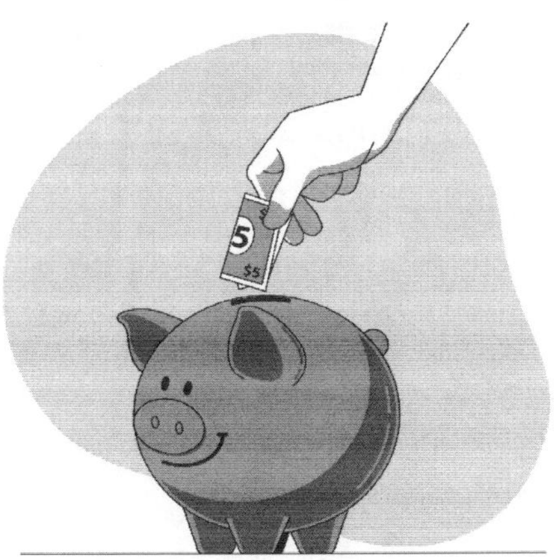

The $5 challenge can also be applied in a positive sense: If you are willing to bet $5 that an answer choice *is* correct, go ahead and mark it as correct.

Summary: Only eliminate an answer choice if you are willing to bet $5 that it is wrong.

Which Answer to Choose

You're taking the test. You've run into a hard question and decided you'll have to guess. You've eliminated all the answer choices you're willing to bet $5 on. Now you have to pick an answer. Why do we even need to talk about this? Why can't you just pick whichever one you feel like when the time comes?

The answer to these questions is that if you don't come into the test with a plan, you'll rely on your impression to select an answer choice, and if you do that, you risk falling into a trap. The test writers know that everyone who takes their test will be guessing on some of the questions, so they intentionally write wrong answer choices to seem plausible. You still have to pick an answer though, and if the wrong answer choices are designed to look right, how can you ever be sure that you're not falling for their trap? The best solution we've found to this dilemma is to take the decision out of your hands entirely. Here is the process we recommend:

Once you've eliminated any choices that you are confident (willing to bet $5) are wrong, select the first remaining choice as your answer.

Whether you choose to select the first remaining choice, the second, or the last, the important thing is that you use some preselected standard. Using this approach guarantees that you will not be enticed into selecting an answer choice that looks right, because you are not basing your decision on how the answer choices look.

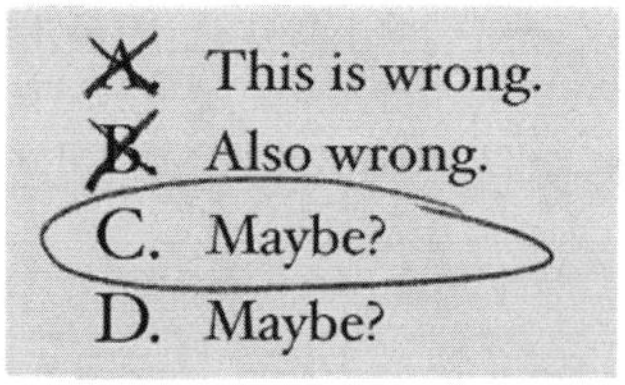

This is not meant to make you question your knowledge. Instead, it is to help you recognize the difference between your knowledge and your impressions. There's a huge difference between thinking an answer is right because of what you know, and thinking an answer is right because it looks or sounds like it should be right.

Summary: To ensure that your selection is appropriately random, make a predetermined selection from among all answer choices you have not eliminated.

Test-Taking Strategies

This section contains a list of test-taking strategies that you may find helpful as you work through the test. By taking what you know and applying logical thought, you can maximize your chances of answering any question correctly!

It is very important to realize that every question is different and every person is different: no single strategy will work on every question, and no single strategy will work for every person. That's why we've included all of them here, so you can try them out and determine which ones work best for different types of questions and which ones work best for you.

Question Strategies

⊘ Read Carefully

Read the question and the answer choices carefully. Don't miss the question because you misread the terms. You have plenty of time to read each question thoroughly and make sure you understand what is being asked. Yet a happy medium must be attained, so don't waste too much time. You must read carefully and efficiently.

⊘ Contextual Clues

Look for contextual clues. If the question includes a word you are not familiar with, look at the immediate context for some indication of what the word might mean. Contextual clues can often give you all the information you need to decipher the meaning of an unfamiliar word. Even if you can't determine the meaning, you may be able to narrow down the possibilities enough to make a solid guess at the answer to the question.

⊘ Prefixes

If you're having trouble with a word in the question or answer choices, try dissecting it. Take advantage of every clue that the word might include. Prefixes can be a huge help. Usually, they allow you to determine a basic meaning. *Pre-* means before, *post-* means after, *pro-* is positive, *de-* is negative. From prefixes, you can get an idea of the general meaning of the word and try to put it into context.

⊘ Hedge Words

Watch out for critical hedge words, such as *likely, may, can, often, almost, mostly, usually, generally, rarely,* and *sometimes.* Question writers insert these hedge phrases to cover every possibility. Often an answer choice will be wrong simply because it leaves no room for exception. Be on guard for answer choices that have definitive words such as *exactly* and *always.*

☑ Switchback Words

Stay alert for *switchbacks*. These are the words and phrases frequently used to alert you to shifts in thought. The most common switchback words are *but*, *although*, and *however*. Others include *nevertheless*, *on the other hand*, *even though*, *while*, *in spite of*, *despite*, and *regardless of*. Switchback words are important to catch because they can change the direction of the question or an answer choice.

☑ Face Value

When in doubt, use common sense. Accept the situation in the problem at face value. Don't read too much into it. These problems will not require you to make wild assumptions. If you have to go beyond creativity and warp time or space in order to have an answer choice fit the question, then you should move on and consider the other answer choices. These are normal problems rooted in reality. The applicable relationship or explanation may not be readily apparent, but it is there for you to figure out. Use your common sense to interpret anything that isn't clear.

Answer Choice Strategies

☑ Answer Selection

The most thorough way to pick an answer choice is to identify and eliminate wrong answers until only one is left, then confirm it is the correct answer. Sometimes an answer choice may immediately seem right, but be careful. The test writers will usually put more than one reasonable answer choice on each question, so take a second to read all of them and make sure that the other choices are not equally obvious. As long as you have time left, it is better to read every answer choice than to pick the first one that looks right without checking the others.

☑ Answer Choice Families

An answer choice family consists of two (in rare cases, three) answer choices that are very similar in construction and cannot all be true at the same time. If you see two answer choices that are direct opposites or parallels, one of them is usually the correct answer. For instance, if one answer choice says that quantity x increases and another either says that quantity x decreases (opposite) or says that quantity y increases (parallel), then those answer choices would fall into the same family. An answer choice that doesn't match the construction of the answer choice family is more likely to be incorrect. Most questions will not have answer choice families, but when they do appear, you should be prepared to recognize them.

☑ Eliminate Answers

Eliminate answer choices as soon as you realize they are wrong, but make sure you consider all possibilities. If you are eliminating answer choices and realize that the last one you are left with is also wrong, don't panic. Start over and consider each choice again. There may be something you missed the first time that you will realize on the second pass.

✓ Avoid Fact Traps

Don't be distracted by an answer choice that is factually true but doesn't answer the question. You are looking for the choice that answers the question. Stay focused on what the question is asking for so you don't accidentally pick an answer that is true but incorrect. Always go back to the question and make sure the answer choice you've selected actually answers the question and is not merely a true statement.

✓ Extreme Statements

In general, you should avoid answers that put forth extreme actions as standard practice or proclaim controversial ideas as established fact. An answer choice that states the "process should be used in certain situations, if..." is much more likely to be correct than one that states the "process should be discontinued completely." The first is a calm rational statement and doesn't even make a definitive, uncompromising stance, using a hedge word *if* to provide wiggle room, whereas the second choice is far more extreme.

✓ Benchmark

As you read through the answer choices and you come across one that seems to answer the question well, mentally select that answer choice. This is not your final answer, but it's the one that will help you evaluate the other answer choices. The one that you selected is your benchmark or standard for judging each of the other answer choices. Every other answer choice must be compared to your benchmark. That choice is correct until proven otherwise by another answer choice beating it. If you find a better answer, then that one becomes your new benchmark. Once you've decided that no other choice answers the question as well as your benchmark, you have your final answer.

✓ Predict the Answer

Before you even start looking at the answer choices, it is often best to try to predict the answer. When you come up with the answer on your own, it is easier to avoid distractions and traps because you will know exactly what to look for. The right answer choice is unlikely to be word-for-word what you came up with, but it should be a close match. Even if you are confident that you have the right answer, you should still take the time to read each option before moving on.

General Strategies

✓ Tough Questions

If you are stumped on a problem or it appears too hard or too difficult, don't waste time. Move on! Remember though, if you can quickly check for obviously incorrect answer choices, your chances of guessing correctly are greatly improved. Before you completely give up, at least try to knock out a couple of possible answers. Eliminate what you can and then guess at the remaining answer choices before moving on.

⊘ Check Your Work

Since you will probably not know every term listed and the answer to every question, it is important that you get credit for the ones that you do know. Don't miss any questions through careless mistakes. If at all possible, try to take a second to look back over your answer selection and make sure you've selected the correct answer choice and haven't made a costly careless mistake (such as marking an answer choice that you didn't mean to mark). This quick double check should more than pay for itself in caught mistakes for the time it costs.

⊘ Pace Yourself

It's easy to be overwhelmed when you're looking at a page full of questions; your mind is confused and full of random thoughts, and the clock is ticking down faster than you would like. Calm down and maintain the pace that you have set for yourself. Especially as you get down to the last few minutes of the test, don't let the small numbers on the clock make you panic. As long as you are on track by monitoring your pace, you are guaranteed to have time for each question.

⊘ Don't Rush

It is very easy to make errors when you are in a hurry. Maintaining a fast pace in answering questions is pointless if it makes you miss questions that you would have gotten right otherwise. Test writers like to include distracting information and wrong answers that seem right. Taking a little extra time to avoid careless mistakes can make all the difference in your test score. Find a pace that allows you to be confident in the answers that you select.

⊘ Keep Moving

Panicking will not help you pass the test, so do your best to stay calm and keep moving. Taking deep breaths and going through the answer elimination steps you practiced can help to break through a stress barrier and keep your pace.

Final Notes

The combination of a solid foundation of content knowledge and the confidence that comes from practicing your plan for applying that knowledge is the key to maximizing your performance on test day. As your foundation of content knowledge is built up and strengthened, you'll find that the strategies included in this chapter become more and more effective in helping you quickly sift through the distractions and traps of the test to isolate the correct answer.

Now that you're preparing to move forward into the test content chapters of this book, be sure to keep your goal in mind. As you read, think about how you will be able to apply this information on the test. If you've already seen sample questions for the test and you have an idea of the question format and style, try to come up with questions of your own that you can answer based on what you're reading. This will give you valuable practice applying your knowledge in the same ways you can expect to on test day.

Good luck and good studying!

Anatomy and Physiology

Cell

A cell is made up of three main parts, the cell membrane, the cytoplasm and the nucleus.

- The jobs of the cell membrane are: To protect the cell; to provide structure for the cell; to transport nutrients into the cell; and transport waste products out of the cell.
- The cytoplasm is made up mostly of water. It is responsible for cellular metabolism. It contains centrosomes, which help with cell division; ribosomes that synthesize proteins; lysosomes that help the cell to digest nutrients; the mitochondria, which produce the cell's energy; Golgi apparatus that combine nutrients; and endoplasmic reticulum, which moves nutrients within the cell.
- The nucleus contains the cell's DNA, which controls the cell's function and also directs proper cellular division.

Respiratory System

The respiratory system is responsible for the intake of air and the exhalation of waste gases. The diaphragm, a large muscle at the base of the sternum, works as an air pump. It alternately pulls air into the lungs, which are located within the thoracic cavity, and expels air from the lungs. Incoming air travels in through the nasal cavities, the pharynx, the larynx, the trachea, and into the lungs. At the top of the lungs, air moves into the bronchi. Bronchi branch into deep bronchioles. Gas exchange takes place in the alveoli, small grape-like sacs in the lungs, where the bloodstream discharges carbon dioxide and takes on oxygen.

External respiration (breathing) involves the inspiration of oxygen and the exhalation of carbon dioxide. Normally, respiration occurs through the nasal cavity. Congested patients or those under exertion breathe through their mouths. Air first passes through the upper respiratory tract (URT), where it is filtered, warmed and humidified: Nares (nostrils); nasopharynx (rear nose); oropharynx (rear mouth); and laryngopharynx (throat). Adenoids and tonsils kill pathogens in the URT. Air then enters the lower respiratory tract (LRT): Larynx (voice box) and vocal chords; trachea (windpipe); right and left bronchi; and lungs. The spongy lungs have a "tree" of bronchioles and tiny, grape-like alveoli clusters, where the exchange of gasses occurs. Carbon dioxide and other waste gases are exhaled. Oxygen from the inhaled breath is carried by red blood cells throughout the body. The diaphragm and muscles of the thoracic wall create the bellows movements necessary for breathing. Mucous in the respiratory system traps invaders, and cilia brush them out. The respiratory system is important for regulating acid-base balance.

Common pathologies that can affect the respiratory system, and that x-ray imaging can be used to diagnose, include: Adult respiratory distress syndrome; asthma;

atelectasis; bronchial adenoma; bronchiectasis; bronchogenic carcinoma; chronic bronchitis; chronic obstructive pulmonary disease; croup; cystic fibrosis; emphysema; histoplasmosis; hyaline membrane disease; Legionnaires' disease; pleural effusion; pneumoconiosis; pneumonia; pneumothorax; pulmonary metastases; and tuberculosis (TB). Each of these diseases or conditions affects the lungs' appearance. When appearance is considered together with other signs and symptoms, it helps doctors to identify a disease (diagnosis), determine how best to treat it, and explain the probable outcome (prognosis).

Review Video: Respiratory System
Visit mometrix.com/academy and enter code: 783075

Gastrointestinal System

GI tract: 6-meter long tube extends from mouth to anus. Upper GI tract: Mouth (buccal mucosa, tongue, and teeth); pharynx; esophagus; and stomach. Lower GI tract: Small intestine (duodenum, jejunum, ileum, and ileocecal valve); and large intestine (ascending, transverse, and descending colon, sigmoid flexure, rectum and anus). The vermiform appendix attaches to the cecum (first section of the ascending colon, closest to the ileocecal valve). The sigmoid flexure leads into the rectum, which terminates in the anus. An internal and an external sphincter control the anus. The GI tract ingests food, digests food, absorbs nutrients and medications, and produce Vitamins B_{12} and K.

Digestive Enzymes Break Down Food

Organ	Chemicals	Food
Salivary glands	Ptyalin	Starch
Stomach	Hydrochloric acid	All
Liver & gall bladder	Bile	Fats
Pancreas	Insulin, glucagon, amylase, & lipase	Sugars & Fats

Common pathologies that can affect the gastrointestinal system, which x-ray imaging can help diagnose, include: Acute cholecystitis (inflamed gallbladder); cancer of the colon, esophagus, stomach, or rectum; cholelithiasis (gallstones); Crohn's disease; diverticulitis; esophageal varices; esophagitis; gastritis; hiatus hernia; ileus; intussusception; irritable bowel syndrome; bowel obstructions; peptic ulcers; pyloric stenosis; ulcerative colitis; and volvulus. Each of these diseases or conditions affects the appearance of the GI system. When considered together with other signs and symptoms, the x-ray image can help doctors identify a disease (diagnosis), determine how best to treat it, and explain the probable outcome (prognosis).

Review Video: Gastrointestinal System
Visit mometrix.com/academy and enter code: 378740

Urinary System

The upper urinary tract consists of two fist-sized, bean-shaped kidneys, each with a kidney pelvis and ureter tube. They lie in the retroperitoneal space, behind the 13th ribs. The lower urinary tract consists of the bladder (behind the symphysis pubis) and the urethra, leading outside the body. The urinary system cleanses the blood, processes waste and some drugs, and eliminates them with excess water as urine. It works with the lungs to regulate the acid-base balance. Blood enters the kidneys through the renal arteries. The kidney tubules filter 150—200 liters of blood daily, screening out nitrogenous waste products (urea, creatinine, and uric acid) and excess water, which flow through the ureters into the bladder. The bladder stores the waste as urine. A sphincter muscle keeps the urine from flowing backwards from the bladder into the kidneys. When the bladder is full enough to trigger the urge to urinate (250 cc—300 cc), the urine exits the body through the urethral meatus.

Common pathologies of the urinary tract that x-ray imaging can help diagnose include: Cancer of the bladder and kidneys; cystitis; glomerulonephritis; polycystic kidney disease; pyelonephritis; renal calculus (kidney stones); urinary reflux and retention; and Wilms' tumor. Each of these diseases or conditions affects the appearance of the urinary tract. When considered together with other signs and symptoms, the x-ray image can help doctors identify a disease (diagnosis), determine how best to treat it, and explain the probable outcome (prognosis).

Review Video: Urinary System
Visit mometrix.com/academy and enter code: 601053

Cardiovascular System

The cardiovascular system is essentially a hydraulic system. It uses a pump, the heart, to move blood throughout the body. The heart is about the size of a fist in an adult, and sits behind the sternum, leaning slightly to the left. The heart is connected to the blood vessels, which are flexible tubes that carry blood. The arteries move oxygenated blood from the heart to all the other organs. Arteries taper into arterioles and then capillaries, which deliver bright red, oxygenated blood to tissues and cells. The capillaries take purplish, deoxygenated blood laden with carbon dioxide and waste products from cells, into venules, and then veins. The blood then makes a return trip through the lungs, where waste gases are removed and the blood receives a new supply of oxygen. It then returns to the heart, where the cycle begins again.

Arteries and arterioles: The arteries and arterioles are the path through which the bright, scarlet red, oxygenated blood travels to reach the body's organs and tissues. There are twenty major arteries in the body and a great network of smaller arterioles. Arterial blood spurts from wounds, because it is under great pressure. By palpating an artery with your fingers, you can take the patient's pulse, to find out the heart rate and if circulation is adequate.

Veins and Venules: When oxygenated blood reaches tissue cells via the capillaries, it passes nutrients and oxygen to the cells. The tissue cells pass waste products and gases to the red blood cells, in turn. The waste-carrying blood turns dark, crimson red, and travels through a system of venules, which expand into large veins, to release the waste gases (mostly carbon dioxide) through the lungs and to receive a fresh supply of oxygen. Venous blood flows gently from wounds. Veins are used to collect blood for testing and to deliver intravenous (IV) medication.

Pulmonary Artery and Pulmonary Vein: Depleted blood reaches the lungs through the pulmonary artery and oxygenated blood travels from the lungs to the heart through the pulmonary vein. This is opposite to the rest of the body, where the arteries carry the oxygen-rich blood and the veins carry the oxygen-poor blood.

Capillaries: These tiny pathways are the smallest part of the cardiovascular system, with a diameter so narrow that blood cells must travel through them single file. The capillaries carry blood directly to tissues and cells, where nutrient/waste exchange takes place. Deoxygenated blood then moves back from capillaries into the larger venules.

The heart is located in the chest cavity between the lungs. It is behind the sternum (breast bone), just a little bit to the left. The heart muscle weighs about a half a pound to a pound. It is a bit larger than a fist. During the average lifespan, a human heart beats more than three and a half billion times — an average of 100,000 beats per day. The heart pumps 2,000 gallons of blood throughout the body each day. The heart is surrounded by the pericardium, a double-walled sac that protects it from rubbing against the ribs. The inner layer is attached to the heart and the outer layer is attached to the diaphragm and the vertebrae. Liquid between the two pericardial layers allows the heart to move while remaining stable. Inside the heart are four chambers. The two smaller, upper chambers are the right and left atria. The larger, lower chambers are the right and left ventricles. The chambers are separated by walls (singular: septum; plural: septa).

The flow of blood within the heart is controlled by four valves: Tricuspid, pulmonary, mitral, and aortic. Bright, scarlet red, oxygen-rich blood flows to the heart from the pulmonary vein into the left atrium. The mitral valve controls that blood as it flows from the left atrium into the left ventricle. The left ventricle is the strongest chamber of the heart. It pumps the blood through the aortic valve out into the body. On the right side of the heart, dark, crimson red, deoxygenated blood moves from the atrium through the tricuspid valve into the right ventricle. Blood from the right ventricle is pumped through the pulmonary valve into the pulmonary artery, where it will travel to the lungs to be re-supplied with oxygen.

The beating of your heart is triggered by electrical impulses. The electrical impulse that causes each contraction builds up in the sinoatrial node (SA). The SA node is found at the top of the right atrium, and is the heart's pacemaker. The SA node is primarily responsible for the heart rate, but other facts can cause the heart rate to change—exertion, stressful situations, and cyclical changes in hormone levels can all have an effect on the heart rate. If the SA node is damaged, any other cell in the heart can become a pacemaker to compensate. The heart will beat automatically even when removed from the chest (automaticity). When the SA node discharges, the electrical impulse travels downwards to the atrioventricular node (AV). It travels down the septum along the Bundle of His. The conduction system splits into two: The right bundle branch (RBB) and the left bundle branch (LBB). The bundles then branch into Purkinje fibers, which contract the heart.

When the heart contracts it pushes blood into the pulmonary artery on the right side and the aorta on the left side. This period of contraction is referred to as systole. During the heart's contraction, the pressure the blood exerts on the artery and vein walls increases throughout the body. When the heart relaxes and dilates, allowing blood to flow into the chambers, it is called diastole. The pressure during the dilation period is lower throughout the body than during the systolic period. Together, these two measures make up the patient's blood pressure (BP). A young adult male has a BP around 120/80 mm/Hg (millimeters of mercury). Most blood pressures are measured at the brachial artery, on the indentation of the inner arm above the elbow. High blood pressure (above 140/90 mm/Hg) is hypertension, which causes blood vessel hardening and damage (atherosclerosis). Low blood pressure (less than 100/60 mm/Hg) indicates hormonal problems, or shock from blood loss, or serious infection.

The heartbeat is triggered by the sinoatrial node, located at the top of the heart. At regular intervals, the SA node sends out an electrical signal that triggers the muscles of the heart to contract. Between the heart's two atria (upper chambers) and the two ventricles (lower chambers) is a nonconductive fatty layer. The ventricles do not contract from the SA signal because it does not reach them. However, when the atria contract they stimulate the atrioventricular node (AV). After a brief delay, it releases a secondary electrical signal, which runs down the Bundle of His, through the left and right bundle branches, and into the Purkinje fibers, which triggers a contraction of the ventricles. This delay and second contraction give the heart its signature, two-part beat (lup-dup, or Korotkoff sounds heard when taking blood pressure).

Nervous System

Nerve endings exist throughout the body, and interconnect in a complex web, to form the peripheral nervous system. They gather sensory inputs (light, sound, temperature, balance, taste, pain, and tactile sensations). The peripheral nervous system conducts all the sensory inputs from the body to the central nervous system, comprised of the brain and spinal cord. The brain decodes and interprets the inputs, and then decides on an appropriate reaction. The brain contains the memory, the decision-making capabilities for the entire body, and the control center for autonomic systems, like digestion, breathing and heart rates.

The nervous system is subdivided into the central nervous system (CNS) and the peripheral nervous system (PNS). The components of the CNS are the brain and spinal cord, in the dorsal cavity. The skull protects the brain, while the vertebrae protect the spinal cord. Meninges are protective membranes insulating the brain and spinal cord. The PNS contains nervous structures outside the dorsal cavity, like long nerves (neuron axons). The PNS is divided into the somatic nervous system and the autonomic nervous system. Somatic nerves control the senses, and body movements that are under conscious, voluntary control. Nerves that control automatic processes, like digestion and breathing, are autonomic. The autonomic nervous system is further divided into the sympathetic nervous system and the parasympathetic nervous system. Sympathetic nerves are involved in the "fight or flight" response from adrenaline, and are activated in times of danger or stress. Parasympathetic nerves are in charge when the individual feels relaxed or is resting from the neurotransmitter acetylcholine.

Lymphatic System

The lymphatic system is comprised of the spleen, thymus, bone marrow, and a series of transparent tubes that run throughout the body, parallel to the blood vessels. The tubes are called lymph vessels, and carry 4 liters of clear lymphatic fluid, or lymph. Lymph circulates throughout the body in the same manner as blood, with valves opening and closing to move the liquid along. There are about 100 small glands, called lymph nodes, stationed at intervals along the lymphatic vessels. The lymphatic fluid carries invaders to the nodes to be destroyed by lymphocytes, a type of white blood cell. Nodes swell during infections. Plasma from the blood vessels seeps out of the capillaries, immerses body tissues, and then drains off into the lymph vessels. Once in the lymphatic system, the plasma is called lymph. Lymph travels through the lymphatic vessels until it reaches the thoracic duct, the largest lymph vessel, extending from L2 to the neck. The lymph drains from the thoracic duct into the blood circulatory system.

Body Habitus

Humans have four main body types (habitus) affecting placement of the diaphragm, stomach, gallbladder, heart, and lungs by 6—8 inches:

- Hypersthenic:
  - 5% of the population; Massive build
  - Broad, deep mid-section; Ribs run almost parallel to the ground
  - Short, wide heart; High diaphragm; Colon frames abdomen
  - High, transverse, medial stomach; High, outside gallbladder
  - Requires more exposures than sthenic
- Sthenic:
  - 50% of the population (average build on which all exposures are based). Fit, strong, athletic, good muscle tone and heavy bone mass
  - Ribs slope at a downward angle; Stomach high and left
  - Evenly spread colon; Gallbladder centered on the right

- Hyposthenic:
    - 35% of the population; More slender than sthenic; Healthy but thin; May be underweight for height; Stomach and gallbladder are high; Requires fewer exposures than the sthenic type
- Asthenic:
    - 10% of the population; Frail, slim, light build; May be unfit and emaciated; Long, shallow, narrow mid-section; Heart is nearly vertical at midline; Low gallbladder, near midline; Low, medial stomach; Low colon; Requires fewest exposures

Main Planes of the Body

The radiologist uses planes to describe body parts in reports to the requisitioning physician. The radiographer uses planes for proper positioning. The four planes are:

- Sagittal: Vertical division into left and right, unequal parts; the body can be divided into an infinite number of parallel planes, all called sagittal planes
- Median sagittal plane: Vertically divides the body equally into left and right halves from the head to toe
- Midcoronal plane: Vertically divides the body into front and rear parts; divides the anterior portion of the body from the posterior.
- Transverse plane: The transverse plan passes through the body horizontally, dividing the upper (superior) body from the lower (inferior); you must state the level of division.

Spinal Topography

The topography of the body is used by the radiographer to ensure correct positioning of the body for an x-ray image. Because people come in all shapes and sizes, the radiographer must memorize basic points of reference and have an understanding of how they correspond to other parts of the body, to adjust the machine appropriately.

The spine has 33 bones: Seven cervical vertebrae (C1—C7); twelve thoracic vertebrae (T1—T12); five lumbar vertebrae (L1—5); five sacral bones (S1—S5); and one coccyx (four tailbones fused together by adulthood). In a physically fit person with normal bones, the vertebrae provide landmarks (points of reference) along the back.

Thoracic (mid-back)

Vertebra	Landmark
T1	2" above the sternal notch
T2—T3 disc space	Sternal notch at the jugular
T4—T5 disc space	Sternal angle
T6—T7 disc space	Lower end of the scapula (midthoracic margin)
T10	Xiphoid tip

The radiographer imagines topographical lines on the patient's body between specific features to make certain the body positioning is proper before capturing an image. Because people come in different shapes and sizes, topographical lines between features help the radiographer customize positioning for the specific patient. Some of the most valuable lines are:

Orbitomeatal Line	Infraorbitomeatal Line	Glabellomeatal Line	Acanthiomeatal Line
Runs between the outer canthus of the eye and the auricular point (the opening of the ear canal)	Runs from below the eye to the auricular point	Runs from the glabella (the space above the nose, between the eyebrows) to the auricular point	Runs from the acanthion (the point where the center of the nose meets the upper lip) to the auricular point

Abdomen

The intersection of the median sagittal plane and the transverse plane divides the abdomen into four quadrants. They are described simply as the right upper quadrant, the right lower quadrant, the left upper quadrant, and the left lower quadrant. These quadrants are used for clinical descriptions. Anatomically speaking, the abdomen is divided into nine regions, like a tic-tac-toe board. The superior or upper three regions are the right hypochondrium, the epigastrium, and the left hypochondrium. The middle three quadrants are the right lumbar, umbilical, and left lumbar. The lower three regions are the right iliac, the hypogastrium, and the left iliac.

Skeletal System

The skeletal system provides a supporting structure for the soft tissues, and protects vital organs and fragile systems. Bone has the strength of cast iron. The skull protects the brain and the sternum protects the heart, for example. The spongy spaces within the bones are filled with marrow. The bone marrow is where the body produces red and white blood cells and platelets. The bone marrow stores calcium so the heart functions correctly. Finally, the bones act as anchors for the muscles and ligaments, which work together with bones to make movement possible. There are five primary types of bones:

1. Long bones like the femur in the thigh
2. Short bones like the carpals in the wrist
3. Flat bones like the ribs
4. Sesamoid bones like the patella in the knee
5. Irregular bones like the vertebrae in the spine

The skeleton can be divided into two major parts. The axial skeleton is made up of all the bones that form the center part of the body, or axis. It is made up of 74 bones, including the skull, the spine, the ribs, and the sternum. Twenty-nine of these bones are in the skull and 33 are in the spine.

The appendicular skeleton is made up of the bones in the extremities. It includes the bones of the arms, legs, pectoral girdle, and pelvic girdle. It also includes the clavicles (collar bones) at the top of the sternum and the scapulae (shoulder blades).

Common pathologies of the skeletal system where x-ray imaging can provide a useful diagnostic tool include: Acromegaly; ankylosing spondylitis; bony cysts; bursitis; bone calluses; clubfoot; congenital hip anomalies; disk herniation; Ewing's sarcoma; fractures; hydrocephalus; giant cell myeloma; gout; multiple myeloma; osteoarthritis; osteoblastic metastases; osteochondroma; osteogenic sarcoma; osteoma; osteogenesis imperfecta; osteomyelitis; osteolytic metastases; osteomalacia; osteopetroses; osteoporosis; Paget's disease; rheumatoid arthritis; rickets; scoliosis; spina bifida; spondylolisthesis; and spondylolysis. Each of these diseases or conditions has a unique effect on the bones, that when taken together with other signs and symptoms, can help doctors identify the disease (diagnosis), determine how best to treat it, and explain the probable outcome (prognosis).

Review Video: <u>Skeletal System</u>
Visit mometrix.com/academy and enter code: 256447

JOINTS

A joint is any area of the body where two or more bones meet. Joints are classified according to their structures, functions, and biomechanical properties.

- Structurally, joints are classified according to the bones that make up the joint and how they are connected: (1) fibrous/immovable, (2) cartilaginous and (3) synovial. Fibrous joints are junctions between bones that are nearly in direct contact, and move very little, e.g., skull sutures. Cartilaginous joints do not have a cavity at the meeting of the bones. They are joined by cartilage and ligaments, and allow for a little movement, e.g., spinal intervertebral disks. Synovial joints move the most. The joints meet in a fibrous capsule lined with a synovial membrane, and connect through ligaments. Knees, elbows, and hips are synovial.
- Functionally, joints are classified by the degree of movement between the bones and are identified as: (1) Synarthrotic, (2) amphiarthrotic and (3) diarthrotic.
- Biomechanically, joints are classified as: (1) simple, (2) compound and (3) complex.

SKULL

The skull, or cranium, is made up of these bones: Frontal, parietal, occipital, temporal, sphenoid, and ethmoid. The squama of the frontal bone is the forehead. The orbital of the frontal bone has the frontal sinuses and the roof of the eye sockets within it. The parietal bones form the sides of the skull. The temporal bones house the auditory structures, including the middle and inner ear. The mandibular fossa (jaw) is also part of the temporal bone, as is the styloid process, where many muscles of the neck are attached. The sphenoid bones are smaller, and located anterior to the temporal bones. The ethmoid bone helps to form the base of the cranium, makes up part of the eye sockets, and the roof of the nose. The occipital bone is the most posterior bone of the cranium (rounded back of the head). The spinal cord enters the skull and connects with the brainstem through the foramen magnum, which is part of the occipital bone.

FACE

The cranium's frontal (forehead) and ethmoid bones create the supporting structure for the facial bones. The bones of the outer face are the: Mandible (lower jaw); maxilla (upper jaw); zygomatic arch (cheek or malar); and vomer (nasal septum). The bones of the inner face are the: Nasal conchae; lacrimals (eye sockets near the nose); L-shaped palatine bones that form the roof of the mouth and nose; and the hyoid, a horseshoe-shaped bone above the styloid process, where tongue muscles and the temporomandibular joint (TMJ) attach. The mandible is the only facial bone able to move.

VERTEBRAL COLUMN

The vertebral column is the pillar that supports the head. It also protects the spinal cord, which is an important part of the central nervous system, and is where the ribs attach. It is a lever for the spinal muscles, allowing the trunk to bend. The neck (cervical) vertebrae are numbered C1—C7. The chest vertebrae (thoracic) are numbered T1—T12. The lower back vertebrae (lumbar) are numbered L1—L5. The back of the pelvis (sacral) is numbered S1—S5. The triangular tailbone (coccyx) is fused in an adult, and has 3—5 separate bones in an infant. When looked at laterally, the cervical vertebrae curve inward, the thoracic vertebrae curve outward, the lumbar curve inward again, and the sacral vertebrae curve outward. Each vertebra has a central mass of bone known as the body, the pedicles of the arch (two columns), a central foramen (space), and several processes (bumps). While they share similar features, the bones in each region of the spine have distinguishing characteristics.

SPINE

The cervical vertebrae have a triangular shape. They are generally smaller than the other vertebrae, although C1 is an exception. C1 is called the atlas because it carries the head. C2 is called the axis because it allows the head to rotate. Vertebrae have natural openings (foramina) where the nerves pass through them. The thoracic vertebrae have facets that allow for rib movements. They are larger than the cervical vertebrae and have more pronounced processes. The lumbar vertebrae are again larger. They are also triangular in shape, which allows them to fit through the pelvis. The sacral vertebrae are longer and narrower than the other vertebrae, a difference that is especially pronounced in males. The sacrum is the fused bones forming the back of the pelvis. The coccyx (tailbone) tapers downwards, and also fuses in adulthood.

Synovial Joints

Synovial joints come in six common varieties. They are hinge joints, pivot joints, saddle joints, ball and socket joints, gliding joints and condyloid joints. A hinge joint allows for movement in a single plane. The elbow is an example of a hinge joint. A pivot joint allows movement around a central axis. The thumb is an example of a saddle joint. A ball and socket joint like the hip allows for a wide range of movements. A gliding joint is the movement among several contiguous bones, like that seen in the ankle or wrist. A condyloid joint allows movement to occur in two directions, but does not allow rotation.

Arms

The upper arm includes: The clavicle (collarbone); scapula (shoulder); the humerus (upper arm); radius and ulna (lower arm); carpals (wrist); metacarpals (hand); and phalanges (fingers). The clavicle wraps around and connects with the scapula. The scapula is triangular in shape. The lateral part of the bone shares a joint with the humerus, the large "funny bone" in the upper arm. Two projections at the distal end of the humerus form the elbow joint with the radius and the ulna, the two bones in the forearm. The radius is on the thumb side, and the ulna is on the little finger side. Between the forearm and the hand, there are eight carpal bones in the wrist. Five metacarpal bones form the structure of the hand. Fourteen phalanges make up the bones in the fingers.

Lower Extremity

The basic structure of the leg includes: The hip (sacrum, ilium); the thigh (femur); the knee (patella); the shin (tibia and fibula); the ankle (tarsals); foot (metatarsals); and toes (phalanges). The hip is joined to the vertebral column through the pelvis, which consists of the ilium, ischium, pubis, and coccyx. The sciatic nerve travels through the greater sciatic notch. The shape of the pelvis differs between the two sexes; females have wide, light pelvis with a larger inlet than males. Their wide pelvis makes many women knock-kneed. The femur is the largest bone in the body; it joins to the hip in a ball-and-socket joint. The distal femur shares a joint with the patella, which also shares a joint with the tibia and the fibula. The ankle and foot bones are similar in structure to the hand, though they have adapted to support the body's weight.

Important Terms

Distal: "Far from." Given a specific point of reference, the distal point is the point farthest from it.

Lateral: Side; away from the middle. The ribs are lateral to the sternum.

Medial: Toward the middle. The sternum is medial to the ribs.

Posterior: Rear or backside of a body part. [However, do not use posterior to describe the backside of the foot (sole), which is ventral.]

Dorsal: Dorsal can be used interchangeably with posterior.

Proximal: "Near to." Given a specific point of reference, a proximal point is nearest to it.

Anterior: Toward the front part of the body or in front of another body part.

Ventral: Belly, chest, palms, and soles. Ventral can also mean the front of any organ. This term can be used interchangeably with anterior, though anterior is the more common term.

Caudal: Away from the head, towards the tail.

Inferior: Under; beneath; structures farther from the head, in relation to other structures.

Central: The middle part of a structure.

Cranial: Closer to the head.

Cephalic: Toward the head.

Superior: Above or toward the head.

Dorsal Recumbent: The patient is lying on his or her back. Supine; also called dorsal decubitus. Dorsal recumbent position is used for most imaging and gynecology.

Ventral Recumbent: The patient is lying face down. Prone; also called ventral decubitus.

Right Lateral Recumbent: The patient is lying on his or her right side. Also called Sim's position, with the arm behind the back and the upper thigh flexed to make vaginal examination easier.

Left Lateral Recumbent: The patient is lying on his or her left side; also called Sim's position.

Projection: The path of the central ray during an imaging procedure.

View: The view refers to the image as it appears to the receptor. It is opposite to the image projection.

Oblique: Slanting or inclined. The term oblique refers to a slanted rotation for a standard position. For example, a patient who is in the right lateral recumbent position but is rolled forward at a slight angle is in an oblique position.

Decubitus Position: Lying down, also called recumbent. Can be supine (dorsal decubitus) or prone (ventral decubitus). Shine the x-ray beam down onto the examination table. For lateral decubitus, position the x-ray gantry laterally to the table so that the beam runs parallel to the floor, to differentiate pleural effusions (where the liquid layers out) from consolidated pneumonia.

RAO: Right Anterior Oblique, a positioning term used by the radiographer to describe a slanted position that brings the right, front part of the body nearer to the film.

LAO: Left Anterior Oblique, when the body is rotated to bring the left, front closest to the film.

RPO: Right Posterior Oblique, a positioning term used by the radiographer to describe an slanted position that brings the right, back part of the body nearer to the film.

LPO: Left Posterior Oblique, when the body is rotated to bring the left, back closest to the film.

Left or Right Lateral Decubitus: An image taken with the patient lying down, on his or her right or left side.

Dorsal Decubitus: An image taken with the patient lying down on his or her back (supine).

Ventral Decubitus: An image taken with the patient lying face down (prone).

Tangential: A type of image taken where the imaging ray merely skims the body part, capturing a profile and preventing superimposition that is typical of most images.

Axial: An image taken with the central ray at a 10° or greater angle to the long axis.

Public Safety in the Health Care Facility

Patient Safety

X-ray technology helps diagnose the extent of an injury or determines pathologies. However, the high voltage of electromagnetic Roentgen rays used in the imaging can cause cancer, burns, and destroy tissues by reducing their blood flow through ionization. A large dose of radiation delivered quickly is more damaging than the identical dose delivered slowly. The radiographer's safe equipment use mitigates the risks, making the benefits of the information gained more important than the risks. The radiographer is responsible for patient, visitor, and staff safety during the procedure. The two most important safety factors are to use the:

1. Minimum number of exposures necessary
2. Smallest amount of radiation needed

In addition to the responsibility held by the radiographer, the patient's physician and radiologist also bear responsibility for only ordering necessary tests and avoiding unnecessary exams.

Ionizing Radiation

X-rays work by transferring photonic energy through tissues. It is possible for the energy to strip electrons within the body, a process called ionization. Ionization causes unstable atoms within the body, which can further damage tissues by "stealing" their electrons. Ionization can also cause new molecules to form, and these foreign molecules are often harmful to the body. Ionization leads to a loss of cellular function. Widespread damage leads to a noticeable decline or change in normal body functions.

There are two types of ionization damage:

1. Damage to cells is somatic damage, and affects only the injured person.
2. Damage to the DNA structure within the cells is genetic damage; if the gonads are involved, subsequent children are also affected.

X-rays are not the only source of ionizing radiation. The radiographer must be aware of various sources of ionizing radiation to ensure the safety of the patient. Ionizing radiation comes from both natural and artificial sources. Environmental sources include natural radiation that is simply present in the atmosphere and always has been. This is called background radiation. Everybody receives is 2 mSv of background radiation annually. The International Commission on Radiological Protection (ICRP) recommends patients receive no more than 1 mSv extra per year. A chest x-ray contributes 0.02 mSv to the patient's overall radiation dose. Radon, which naturally occurs in the earth, is the greatest source of exposure to ionizing radiation. Natural sources make up 82% of average human exposure. Artificial or man-made radiation makes up the other 18%. Artificial exposure comes from diagnostic imaging, small amounts of radiation found in some consumer products, and the dispersed radiation in the atmosphere from nuclear testing.

Photoelectric Interactions, Compton's Interaction, and Coherent Scatter

Photoelectric interactions occur when an x-ray photon strikes the K-shell of an atom. The energy from the photon is transferred to the K-shell electron, stripping the electron from the atom. The photon loses all its energy and is gone. The electron continues to move among other atoms, potentially causing further ionization. The disrupted K-shell may also release low-energy photons.

Compton's interaction is similar, but the x-ray photon does not lose all its energy. Instead, it moves on at a different angle (scattered) and with less energy.

Coherent scatter occurs when low-energy photons are used. This causes atoms to vibrate, but not to lose electrons. The vibrating atomic electrons release energy equal to that received from the photons, but in a different direction.

Appropriate Radiation Exposure and Absorbed Doses

Traditional radiation measures in the USA are roentgens, rads, rems, and curies. However, the National Institute of Standards and Technology discourages the use of rads. Since 1970, NIST encourages the Système Internationale (SI) term, gray (Gy), for absorbed doses.

Two main factors to consider during x-ray testing are the amount of radiation:

1. Exposure due to proximity to the radiation source
2. Absorbed by the patient

Calculate radiation exposure as 1 R (roentgen) per kilogram of air in the room. Patients' radiation doses are measured in millisieverts (mSv); a chest x-ray delivers 0.02 mSv. Generally, most x-ray procedures result in 1 rad per gram of exposed tissue, in traditional measurement.

To help ensure patient safety, the National Council on Radiation Protection and Measurement (NCRP), the International Commission on Radiologic Protection, and the Nuclear Regulatory Commission set standards for safe absorbed doses of radiation. The limits set are meant to ensure that there is little risk of somatic or genetic damage from ionization. These organizations encourage radiographers to use the lowest reasonable dose to achieve reasonably accurate diagnostic results. The NCRP recommends that occupational exposure be limited annually to 5 rems and that lifetime exposure be limited to an average of 1 rem a year. For people undergoing procedures frequently, annual exposure should be limited to 0.1 rem. For people undergoing rare procedures, an annual limit of .5 is recommended. For exposure that keeps to the skin, eyes and extremities, an annual limit of 5 rems is the standard. An embryo or fetus should not be exposed to more than .5 rems during gestation and not more than .05 rems per month.

The radiographer determines the amount of exposure and the quality of the diagnostic image by calculating these exposure factors:

1. The best kVp level for the area of the body being x-rayed
2. The optimum level of mAs

By setting these both to optimal levels, the radiographer can reduce exposure without compromising accuracy. To determine optimum levels, the radiographer uses calipers to measure the area to be exposed. He or she also consults a technique chart, and uses automatic exposure controls.

The film-screen processing can affect the time of exposure. Faster film-screen combinations mean less radiation. However, different body parts may require slower combinations for accuracy. Use the fastest combination possible that will still provide accurate results.

Grids

Using a grid can increase the accuracy of a procedure, and potentially can reduce long-term patient exposure by reducing repeat procedures. However, use extreme care, because taking a grid radiograph does require a higher level of radiation. The radiographer must be certain to use the correct type of grid and the proper ratios for the area of the body being examined.

Repeat procedures are necessary when accurate results are not achieved during the first procedure. Repeating a procedure increases the patient's exposure, so it is always desirable to avoid repeat procedures. If the radiographer must repeat a procedure, he or she must document the reasons for the repeat. Radiology supervisors monitor discarded film to track how often repeats occur. Should a radiographer show a pattern of frequent repeats, additional education may be ordered by the supervisor.

Cell Damage

Young cells are more prone to damage than mature cells. Cells in the process of dividing are most sensitive to radiation and its damaging effects. Cells that contain a high amount of oxygen at the time of exposure are also more sensitive. Cells that are fully matured or cells that have specialized to perform a specific function are less likely to be damaged by radiation. Radiation can temporarily lower the number of red blood cells. Epithelial tissues, cells that form a lining around many of the body's organs, are highly sensitive to radiation, and so are reproductive cells. Muscle cells and nerve tissues are resistant to radiation damage.

ALARA

ALARA means "As Low as Reasonably Achievable." It refers to using the lowest dose of radiation possible to achieve reliable results. The radiographer can do these things to increase reliability, making it possible to use lower doses of radiation:

- Take a thorough patient history. Understand how often the patient has undergone radiographic procedures in the past, especially in recent history.
- Open lines of communication with your patient and his or her caregiver. Clearly communicate instructions to help procedures go safely and smoothly; get a translator or assistant, if necessary.
- Properly immobilize the patient to limit the need for repeated exposures

Too much radiation damages the patient's cells and the DNA. Doses required for this kind of damage are much higher than those that used in diagnostics, but the implications are important for the radiographer to understand. Somatic damage can manifest as a depressed blood cell count for all types of blood cells, or as a disruption in gastrointestinal function, or in failure of the central nervous system. All can result in death. Cancer, cataracts, and thyroid damage are also possible side effects. Damage to DNA will cause mutations that pass from parent to child. Often, these mutations affect recessive genes, causing recessive defects to present, which would not have presented otherwise.

Gonadal Shields

Genetic damage is one of the risks of radiation exposure and reproductive cells are especially prone to damage from radiation exposure. A gonadal shield can be used to protect reproductive cells from damage and should be used whenever possible. A lead gonadal shield reduces female ovary exposure by 50%, and male testicular exposure by 95%. The two most common types of shields are flat contact shields and shadow shields. The flat contact shield is a flat piece of lead (usually flexible) that is laid over the gonads. A shadow shield is placed in the field of the beam within the housing of the x-ray machine. It shields the gonads without requiring contact with the patient.

Whenever the gonads are within 0.5 centimeter or less of the range of the primary beam, the radiographer should provide a gonadal shield to protect the patient. A gonadal shield is especially important if the patient is young or within childbearing years. There may be situations when gonadal shielding will interfere with the procedure. In those situations, it is acceptable for the radiographer to forgo using the gonadal shield.

Automatic Exposure Control

Most instruments have the option to use automatic exposure control or to set a manual timer. The AEC works by automatically shutting off when the desired optical density for the radiograph has been reached. When using the automatic control during a low kilovoltage examination, the radiographer should be aware that the AEC could fail during these kinds of images. To safeguard the patient from unnecessary exposure, the radiographer should set the manual timer for 2 seconds to make sure the machine stops exposure when it should. A mammogram is an example of the kind of procedure where the AEC may fail to terminate when it should. No matter what type of timer your instrument uses, check it periodically to ensure that it is performing accurately, as a simple safety precaution.

Positioning

Proper positioning is important for safety-related reasons. First and foremost, proper positioning helps to render an accurate result the first time. By taking care to position the area to be x-rayed, the radiographer can reduce the number of repeat images needed, thus reducing the patient's overall exposure:

1. Ensure the body part is on the cassette and positioned in a way that will make an image of the desired features possible
2. Be certain that the area in question is aligned properly

Image the long axis of the body part in the same direction as the long axis of the film

Exposure Techniques

In most situations, the radiographer can refer to technique charts to determine the optimal radiographic techniques to use for a specific procedure. However, in some circumstances, the radiographer will need to make adjustments to the techniques used:

- Some pathological conditions will require adjustments in order to capture an accurate, useful image
- Patients who are very young or very old may require different exposure techniques
- Some imaging conditions are not ideal and require adjustments, such as mobile radiography and cross-table projections
- Depending on the patient's habitus, the radiographer may have to make additional adjustments of 6—8 inches for the heart, lungs, stomach, intestines, liver, and gallbladder

Staff Radiation Exposure

In addition to protecting the patient during a radiograph, the radiographer must also consider his or her safety and the safety of attending staff. The primary source of exposure for the staff is scattered radiation. Reduce radiation by properly collimating the beam and by using a fast film-speed combination. Use lead aprons, keep an adequate distance from the x-ray tube, and stay behind a protective barrier during the procedure. Such a barrier is 1/16th inch lead equivalent, meaning it gives the same protection as that thickness of lead. For example, if you stand unprotected 1 cm—2cm in front of the window, and the x-ray tube is operating at 40,000 V and 25 mA, the 1 kW of power the machine generates will cause incurable third degree burns to exposed parts of your body. Radiographers who use portable radiography machines, fluoroscopy machines, and surgical radiography machines are at additional risk of exposure. Pay greater attention to reducing exposure using portable units.

Children

It is important that the radiographer recognize the unique challenges that a child presents. Some children will have difficulty being still. Some will be frightened. Others may be uncooperative. First, the radiographer makes a personal introduction to both the child and parents. The radiographer must be friendly and positive with the child, and address explanations to both the parents and child. The radiographer watches the parents for cues as to how involved they need to be. Once the child understands what will happen, the radiographer determines if the child must be immobilized, and the best way to do that. The radiographer should work with the radiologist to determine proper exposures and safety procedures. Finally, if there are any signs of child abuse, the radiographer must report them. If you need help to find your local number to report abuse, call Childhelp at 1-800-4-A-CHILD (1-800-422-4453), then push 1 to talk to a hotline counselor.

Trauma Victims

The first "Golden Hour" after the accident is critical for trauma victims. Most die of hypoxia and hypoventilation. Blunt injuries require portable chest x-rays in Resuscitation with the patient supine, and slightly over-penetrated films to visualize the thoracic spine and aorta. Puncture wounds require the patient sitting up to visualize all entry and exit wounds, and to detect pneumothorax, left hemothorax, and diaphragm injury. Penetrating trauma patients deteriorate faster than blunt trauma patients, but recover quicker.

The trauma radiographer is adept at positioning and exposure, quick and accurate to capture the diagnostic images the doctors need:

- Remain calm to avoid mistakes.
- Do not move your patient in a way that causes additional injury or exacerbates existing injuries. Seek assistance to move him or her to the x-ray table. Allow your patient to help with movements as much as he or she is capable.
- Use the correct personal protective equipment (PPE) for body fluids.
- Clear communication with your patient is important for getting a good quality image.

Scheduling Considerations

Often, radiographic tests require the patient to undergo a sequence of procedures. The radiographer must review the patient's history and estimate the patient's condition and strength. When possible, schedule the patient to complete several required procedures in a single day, to cut down on the patient's travel time. However, if the patient's health or financial situation makes such an arrangement difficult, schedule procedures to provide the maximum level of comfort possible without compromising the level of care. The radiographer should accommodate these patients with morning appointments: Diabetics; fasting patients who cannot eat until after their procedure; and young children who require naps and frequent feedings. Remain attuned to patient needs and be as flexible as possible in accommodating those needs.

Patient History

The patient's history should provide the radiographer with detailed information about the:

- Suspected or existing injury or pathology targeted for x-ray examination
- Patient's range of motion
- Pre-existing medical conditions that may affect the test (e.g., diabetes, arthritis, emphysema)

After reviewing the existing history, the radiographer questions the patient and caregiver to verify:

- The patient's injury or pathology
- Any limitations to movement the patient is experiencing
- How and when the injury occurred or onset of the pathology
- How much pain the patient is experiencing and where
- If the patient experiences any numbness, weakness or tingling
- If there are other significant signs and symptoms, like heart problems, fever, nausea, or shortness of breath

Finally, if the patient and caregiver cannot communicate clearly, the radiographer should phone the doctor's office to clarify the purpose of ordering the exam.

Intentional Misconduct

Intentional misconduct can result in a civil suit. While these forms of misconduct are called intentional, which makes them sound like they would be obvious and easy to avoid, it is important that the radiographer understand them so that misunderstandings can be avoided.

- Assault occurs when a patient is afraid of being injured.
- Battery includes inappropriate touching, harm that results from the radiographic procedure, or radiographic procedures done incorrectly.
- False imprisonment includes holding an individual against his will. Individuals who must be restrained during a procedure need to clearly understand what will happen and provide their consent prior to application of the restraints.
- An invasion of privacy suit can be brought if confidential information is not handled with the proper care. In most cases, good communication between the radiographer and the patient, with the radiographer consistently acting in a considerate manner, can protect the radiographer from intentional misconduct suits.

Unintentional Misconduct

Unintentional misconduct includes neglect that results in substandard care, gross negligence that puts the patient at direct risk of harm, and contributory negligence, where the radiographer's actions contribute to the risk of injury. Unintentional misconduct is based on a doctrine of reasonable prudence. This means if the radiographer takes all actions to ensure proper care that a reasonable person could expect her to take, then negligence did not exist. If the radiographer is properly trained, takes proper care to learn the history of the patient, communicates clearly to with the patient, and performs the procedures up to the standard of her training, then she should be safe from accusations of negligence.

Malpractice

To establish whether or not malpractice has occurred, four conditions are examined:

1. Is there an established standard of care? This means that the radiographer can be reasonably expected to know what is expected, as far as care and procedure is concerned.
2. Did the radiographer violate established standards of care in some way?
3. Was the injured party indeed injured, and suffered either a loss or an injury due to the radiographer's failure to meet established standards of care?
4. Finally, can the loss or damages be proven to have been caused by the radiographer's negligence?

All four of these conditions must be met for a finding of malpractice.

Chart Notations

A patient's chart provides a legal health record, and is a subpoenable court document. It outlines the patient's reason for seeking the current procedure, and what steps have been taken in that procedure. When a radiographer writes in the patient's chart, it is referred to as charting. Charting practices vary, depending on the place of employment, so the radiographer must understand the standard practices his particular employer expects. Handwritten chart notes must be in indelible ink, preferably black or blue. Many healthcare organizations require computerized notes. When charting, the radiographer must clearly state: The patient's condition; names of the procedures; any patient reactions that occur; name and dose of any substance administered orally or by injection; date and time. The radiographer must sign the chart notations. Include any chain-of-custody and release of information forms in the chart, and ensure they are properly witnessed.

Patient Transfer Procedures

When a patient arrives in Radiology from another part of the hospital:

1. Check the patient's ID bracelet to ensure the name matches the chart and requisition, and that the correct patient is being transferred.
2. If the patient is conscious, coherent, and understands a language you speak fluently, ask for his or her name and birth date for additional confirmation.

3. Double check the identity of the patient with the porter, and be certain it matches the records.
4. Introduce yourself to the patient and caregiver.
5. Clearly explain to the patient and caregiver what you are going to do.
6. When lifting a patient, keep bent knees and a straight back. Get an assistant and use a bed lift to help move heavy patients.
7. If the patient needs oxygen, or has an IV, or other equipment attached, ensure a nurse who knows the patient remains for the procedure.
8. Keep communication open to avoid misunderstandings and calm the patient.

Moving Patients

To move a patient safely from a wheelchair onto an x-ray table:

Situate the wheelchair so it is parallel to the long side of the x-ray table. Set the wheelchair brakes. Have a step stool equipped with a handle ready for the patient to use. Stand in front of the wheelchair facing the patient. Help the patient to stand up out of the wheelchair. The patient uses the stool and the radiographer's shoulder for balance. After the patient steps up onto the stool, the radiographer helps him to pivot, so that his back is to the table. From here, the patient should be able to slide into a sitting position on the edge of the table. Depending on the patient's level of mobility, the radiographer may need to place an arm behind the patient's shoulders and under the patient's knees, to help the patient move into the proper position for the procedure.

When a procedure is completed, the radiographer must assist the patient back to the wheelchair. A nonambulatory (a patient who is not able to walk) will need the most assistance. First, the radiographer brings the wheelchair close and parallel to the x-ray table. The radiographer firmly engages the wheelchair brakes. The radiographer helps the patient to sit up on the x-ray table, and allows the patient time to adjust to the new position to avoid sudden hypotension. Once the patient is ready, the radiographer faces the patient. The radiographer reaches both arms around the patient, placing his hands on the patient's scapulae. The radiographer gently assists the patient into a standing position. While still supporting the patient, the radiographer helps him to pivot, so that the backs of his legs are against the wheelchair. Finally, the radiographer gently assists the patient into a sitting position in the chair, and then makes sure the patient is situated comfortably and is covered modestly.

Moving a patient from a cart to the x-ray table requires more than one person. At least two people, and preferably three or four, are needed to execute a smooth transfer. Position a draw sheet under the patient to help with the transfer. If there are only two people, one is responsible for supporting the patient's neck and shoulders, and the other supports the pelvis and knees. The two people moving the patient should communicate, so that they lift and move the patient in a coordinated, smooth motion. If additional people are available to help, they should support the patient at each side. Ensure that IV lines and monitor cords do not entangle the patient. Rearrange clothing to protect the patient's modesty and preserve warmth.

Infection Transmission

Infection is commonly transmitted through:

- Direct person-to-person contact: Impetigo, athlete's foot, warts, touching syphilis chancres (rare)
- Iatrogenic transmission: MRSA; aspergillosis; hepatitis from infected blood products
- Airborne: Measles, Tuberculosis, Chickenpox
- Droplets released during sneezing and coughing: Mumps, Pertussis, Influenza
- Foodborne or waterborne infections (fecal/oral route): Salmonella, Norwalk, Campylobacter; E. coli 0157:H7
- Animal to human transfer: Malaria from mosquitoes; Lyme disease from ticks; Chagas disease from triatomine bugs; leishmaniasis and plague from rodents.
- Indirect contact with a fomite (infected surface): Lice from hairbrushes; rotavirus from diapers; Legionnaire's disease from air conditioning reservoir.

Standard or universal precautions mean healthcare workers control the spread of disease by assuming every patient is infectious.

Your employer must provide:

- A safety officer who trains all Radiology personnel in correct procedures
- Free PPE (lab coats, gloves, face shields, plastic aprons, shoe covers and goggles); and must clean and maintain it
- Written policies for handling and discarding tissue and waste

Your responsibilities:

- Wash your hands frequently; Wear correct PPE
- Handle and dispose of contaminated equipment, tissues, and blood in a way that controls the spread of pathogens
- Refrain from eating, drinking or smoking in Radiology
- Do not store food in refrigerators that contain contrast dyes, medications, or other biological material
- Decontaminate Radiology work surfaces with hypochlorite at regular intervals and whenever a spill occurs
- Follow proper aseptic technique to protect your patient from surgical infection when working in O.R. If you suspect any patient has a contagious disease, isolate him/her and notify Infection Control immediately. Check your Radiology lab's written procedures; follow OSHA standards.

Medical Emergencies

The radiographer must anticipate and recognize an emergent situation and react appropriately. Common emergencies in Radiology include: Anaphylaxis (allergic reaction to contrast dyes or radiology medications, like adenosine); burns from new tattoo ink or indwelling metal; epileptic seizure; cardiac arrest; respiratory distress;

severe bleeding and shock in trauma patients. The radiographer must have prior training in first aid, CPR, the use of an EpiPen, emergency tracheotomy procedure, and oxygen administration. Post the number to call for the Code Blue team or EMS beside your phone, according to your employer's policy. After emergency personnel have been called, begin CPR or first aid, as required. Know the nearest crash-cart's location, and familiarize yourself with its contents. If a patient goes into shock, move the patient into a recumbent position and cover with a warmed blanket. If the patient could aspirate, roll towels to keep the patient in recovery position. Take the patient's blood pressure and administer oxygen as needed. Try to handle the situation away from view of your other patients.

Support Equipment

In many circumstances, the radiographer performs procedures on a patient who is using support equipment. Examples of support equipment include: Ventilators; nasogastric tubes; chest tubes; intravenous medication equipment (bags, tubing, and pain pumps); urinary catheters; and oxygen cylinders. In most cases, the radiographer must not remove the equipment during the procedure. Tubes must not be dislodged, pinched, or bent, as the flow of liquid or gas will stop. If a tube is disturbed, the radiographer should call for appropriate assistance. Always try to have a nurse who knows the patient attend the procedure, and accompany the patient back to his/her unit.

Contrast Media

Media, such as air, iodine and barium, help to create a better diagnostic image. Contrast media can be ingested or injected. In all cases, the radiographer must check the patient's history for suspected or known sensitivity to the contrast media in question. If the patient has sensitivity, the contrast agent should not be used. Gadolinium and iodine-based contrasts are the most toxic to the kidneys, and effects can develop 3 months after imaging. Anaphylaxis is immediate and life threatening.

Some patients will have an adverse reaction to contrast media even if it has never been administered before. The radiographer must be alert for: Flushing; hives; nausea; low blood pressure; irregular heartbeat; sneezing; heat sensations; itching; disorientation; convulsions; and dyspnea (difficulty breathing). Always have a crash cart nearby that is stocked with: An EpiPen; antihistamines; saline and D5W IV bags; three 50 ml ampoules of sodium bicarbonate; 200 mg theophylline; a tracheostomy kit; oxygen; and an automated external defibrillator (AED).

Prior to injecting a patient with an iodinated contrast medium, check for previous reactions or known sensitivities. Diabetics stop taking metformin 48 hours before the test, and only resume taking it after the lab returns normal kidney function results. Beware nephrotoxicity in patients with: Congestive heart failure; pulmonary edema; serum creatinine >120 mm/L; intra-arterial balloons; anemia; systole <80 mm/Hg; and aged >75 years. Use less than 100 ml of iso-osmolar, nonionic contrast media, if possible. Explain possible reactions to the patient. Note baseline information, such as normal skin tone, heart rate, the tone and pitch of the patient's voice, and anxiety levels. After the injection, ask the patient questions. Making her talk will help you determine if there is any change in the patient's voice, which can indicate swelling of the larynx. Other than stepping to the control panels to take an image, remain with the patient at all times after the injection to monitor for any signs of a reaction.

Hazardous Materials Disposal

Many chemicals used in the Radiology lab are dangerous if inhaled, swallowed, or absorbed through the skin. Sheets, towels and instruments contaminated with blood, urine, feces, wound drainage, amniotic fluid, vaginal secretions, semen, sweat, tears, saliva, and CSF are biohazards. Proper handling and disposal of such materials is a job requirement under federal law (OSHA). Ask your Safety Officer for the safety data sheets (SDS) that describe the proper handling and disposal of the hazardous substances you use, read them, and keep them readily available. Chemicals must be clearly labeled and properly stored. Ask the Safety Officer and Infection Control practitioner about which personal protective equipment (PPE) to wear for chemicals and biohazards. The US Department of Labor's Occupational Health and Safety Administration has a Web site at http://www.osha.gov that provides important updates you are required to adopt as part of your standards of practice.

Important Terms

Primary radiation: When the radiation leaves the x-ray tube, it is primary radiation.

Exit radiation: The x-rays move through the soft tissue, scattering and reflecting, depending on the density of the materials they strike. Some of the radiation passes completely through the patient and is captured as the image used in diagnostics. This is called exit radiation.

Attenuation: As the x-rays pass through the patient, they are absorbed and scattered, depending on the density of the different tissues they strike. The loss of intensity during this process is called attenuation.

Heterogeneous beam: An x-ray beam that contains photons of many varying energy levels.

Fundamentals of Electricity, Electronics, and Solid-state Devices

Fractions

Fractions represent equal parts of a whole number. Fractions have a numerator (the number of parts) over a denominator (the total number of parts to make one whole). An improper fraction has a numerator that is greater than the denominator. When adding fractions, the numerators are simply added together. The denominators must be equal. When denominators are different, use the following process to find a common denominator:

$$a/x + b/y = ay/xy + bx/xy = (ay + bx)/xy$$

When two fractions are multiplied, the numerators are multiplied together and the denominators are multiplied together, as follows:

$$a/x \text{ X } b/y = ab/xy$$

When dividing fractions, the second fraction is inverted and then the two are multiplied, as follows:

$$a/x \div b/y = a/x \text{ X } y/b = ay/xb$$

Significant Figures

When calculating a mathematical equation, it is often necessary for the radiographer to round the number appropriately. Significant numbers help determine how many decimals to round to, so as to provide the correct amount of precision. In essence, the answer should only be as precise as the least precise number in the problem. When adding or subtracting numbers, round the answer to the same decimal place as the number with the fewest digits past the decimal point. In multiplication or division, the answer should have the same number of significant figures as the number within the problem that has the fewest. In division, numbers to both the right and left of the decimal point count as significant. In the problem 3.082 X 7.32, the answer, 22.56024, should be rounded to 22.6 to reflect three significant figures.

Solving Algebraic Problems

Algebraic problems involve an unknown variable. The known numbers are manipulated through multiplication, division, addition, and subtraction to determine the value of the unknown number. The unknown number is usually depicted as a letter, often x, y, or z. For example the problem is stated as, "Find x." If the unknown, x, is multiplied by a known number, divide both sides of the equation by that number to determine x, as in:

If $ax = b$, then $x = b/a$.

If a number is added to x, as in x + a = b, then subtract a from both sides of the equation, so that x + a – a = b – a or x = b – a, since a – a would be zero.

If an equation is in fraction form, such as a/x = b/c, then use cross-multiplication to solve for x. In other words ac = bx, so x = ac/b.

Numbering Systems

The standard number system is based on the number ten. When expressed in fraction form, whole numbers are the familiar 1, 10, 100, 1,000, 10,000, etc. Numbers less than one are expressed as a numerator and denominator, such as 1/10, 1/100, etc. When expressed in decimal form, the whole numbers are the same. The numbers less than one are written to the right of the decimal point, such as 0.1, .01, .001, etc. When written in exponential form, the base number is raised to a power to express larger numbers. 100 is 10^2, for example. Numbers less than one are raised to a negative power. For example, .01 is 10^{-2}. This is referred to as scientific notation and is commonly used in radiography. The logarithmic form of numbers uses the exponent as the number, rather than a base number raised to a power. So, 1,000 becomes 3.000 when expressed as a log using base 10.

Units of Measure

The radiographer has several concerns: The intensity of radiation coming from the x-ray machine; the dose absorbed by the patient; the exposure of the professionals working in the office; and the radioactivity of the materials that produce the x-ray radiation.

The intensity of radiation exposure is measured with a unit called the roentgen (R), which measures the electric charge per unit mass of air. Most x-ray machines are set to milliroentgen (mR). The absorbed dose of radiation by the patient is measured in terms of rads, or Radiation Absorbed Dose. Occupational exposure and environmental exposure is measured in rems. A rem is used to measure overall exposure from different kinds of radiation. The curie is used to measure the amount of actual radioactive material.

Mechanics

Mechanics is the branch of physics that studies the motion of objects. Physicists use vectors to describe the motion of an object. A vector describes both the direction of motion and the magnitude of the motion. In simpler terms, motion is often described as velocity and or acceleration. Velocity is the amount of distance an object covers in a certain amount of time. Acceleration is how much the velocity changes within a timeframe.

Isaac Newton discovered three laws of motion.

- Law of inertia—objects at rest tend to stay at rest and objects in motion tend to stay in motion unless acted on by external forces.
- Law of force — the force on an object equals the object's mass multiplied by the acceleration the force causes.
- Law of reactions — for every action there is an equal and opposite reaction.

Half-Life

Some atoms have an unstable nucleus. To achieve stability, these atoms will spontaneously emit particles. The loss of particles will eventually transform the atom into another type of atom, in a process called radioactive decay. For stability, the atom's protons and neutrons must be in the proper ratio. This means the number of neutrons (which determine an atom's isotope) is very important to whether an atom will be radioactive or not. It is possible to use particle accelerators or nuclear reactors to create radioactive isotopes of certain atoms, such as barium. During the process of radioactive decay, a particle typically releases alpha particles, beta particles, and gamma rays. Radioactive materials decay at a consistent rate measured by the half-life, the amount of time it takes for the amount of radioactive material to be reduced by half.

Electromagnetic Spectrum

Photons are massless particles of electromagnetic energy. There is a wide range of energy levels along the electromagnetic spectrum. People are most familiar with the visible light spectrum. Most animals have developed organs to detect different ranges of the electromagnetic spectrum. Humans can perceive short wavelengths (violet) up to longer wavelengths (red) of electromagnetic energy. This is the visible light spectrum. Invisible parts of the electromagnetic spectrum at higher energy than violet light are ultraviolet, x-ray and gamma ray radiation. Infrared, microwaves, and radio wave have longer wavelengths than red light.

Radiolucency and Inverse Square Law

Radiolucency: Radiolucent materials allow x-rays to pass through with some attenuation. Radiopaque materials are too dense to allow x-rays to pass through.

Inverse Square Law: As light travels away from its source, its intensity decreases quickly. The further it travels, the lower its intensity becomes. The rate of fall of the intensity is inversely proportional to the distance traveled. This relationship is called the inverse square law.

The basic physics behind taking an x-ray involve the energy of the x-rays striking radiolucent tissues and passing through to be captured on an image receptor.

Piezoelectric Effect, Thermoelectric Effect, and Photoelectric Effect

Certain nonconductive materials, like quartz crystals or Rochelle salt, create a measurable effect when pressure is applied to them. A charge separation occurs that can be measured as a voltage across the material. This effect depends on the angle of the crystal. It is called the piezoelectric effect and can be used to create a transducer.

When two wires made of different metals are joined in a coil, there are two junctions where the metals meet. The temperature difference across the two junctions can be measured in terms of voltage. This is the thermoelectric effect.

Certain materials, like selenium and silicon, generate an electric current when exposed to light. The photoelectric effect can be used to measure the light's intensity and exposure or light absorption.

Frequency

The frequency of the x-ray beam describes its energy. It is possible for x-rays to have differing frequencies. To determine the x-ray's frequency, you must know the x-ray's wavelength. The x-ray's frequency is the speed of light divided by the x-ray's wavelength. The speed of light is constant at 3×10^8 m/s.

If the wavelength of an x-ray is 4.3×10^{-11} m, then the frequency is 3×10^8 m/s divided by 4.3×10^{-11} m. The frequency is 6.97×10^{18} Hz.

If the frequency is known, it is possible to determine the wavelength in the same fashion.

To determine an x-ray's energy in electron Volts requires the use of Planck's quantum equation, which states that energy is equal to Planck's constant X the frequency. The value of Planck's constant is 4.15×10^{-15} electron Volt seconds (eVs). If an x-ray beam is known to have energy of 7.5×10^4 electron Volts (eV), the frequency can be determined by dividing the energy by Planck's constant.

In this example, the equation would be 7.5×10^4 eV / 4.15×10^{-15} eVs. The result is 1.8×10^{19} Hz. (Hertz are measured in cycles/second.)

Photonic Energy

Planck's quantum equation can be used to determine an x-ray's (or other electromagnetic source's) energy if the frequency is known. The equation used is $E = hf$, where E is energy measured in electron Volts, h is Planck's constant (4.15×10^{-15} eVs), and f is the frequency measured in Hz. If electromagnetic radiation has a frequency of 640 kHz, then the energy is:

$E = 4.15 \times 10^{-15}$ eVs x 6.4×10^5 Hz. Hertz is measured as cycles/second or s^{-1}, so the result is 2.66×10^{-9} eV.

Energy Equivalence

Unlike photons, electrons have mass. This means that a different process is used to determine the energy equivalence of an electron. In other words, if the electron's mass were to be converted to pure energy, how much energy would result? To determine the energy equivalence of mass, Einstein's equation is used: $E = mc^2$ where E is energy, m is mass, and c is the constant speed of light. An electron's mass is very small: 9.109×10^{-31} kilograms. The energy equivalence of an electron would then be $9.109 \times 10^{-31} \times (3 \times 10^8)^2$. The resulting energy in joules is 8.1972×10^{-14}. Joules can be converted to eV by multiplying by 6.24×10^{18} eV/J.

Electrostatic Charges

Static electricity, the buildup of a charge on an object due to friction, is measured in coulombs. One coulomb is equal to 6.24×10^{18} electron charges. The charge from a single electron is much too small to provide a useful measurement, so coulombs are used, instead.

Milliampere-seconds are one of the settings that radiographers control on the imaging system. Amperes are a measure of coulombs per second, so milliampere-seconds are actually a measure of millicoulombs, or the measure of the electrostatic charge.

The size of electrostatic force is described by Coulomb's law, which states that the force (F) is equal to a constant (k) multiplied by the size of the two electrostatic charges that are interacting (Q_A and Q_B) and divided by the square of the distance between the charges (r).

Ohm's Law

Ohm's law is used to describe the relationship between the current, electric potential, and resistance of a circuit. The resistance of a circuit will be equal to its electric potential divided by the current. Resistance is measured in ohms, electric potential is measured in volts, and electric current is measured in amperes. If any two of these factors are known, the third can be determined using this equation.

For example, if the voltage across a conductor is measured at 3 V when a .4-ampere current is flowing through the conductor, what is the resistance of the conductor? Using Ohm's law, the resistance will equal 3V divided by .4 A. The resistance of the conductor is 7.5 ohms.

Series Circuit

In a circuit that is wired in series, all the elements of the circuit are connected in a linear fashion across the circuit. In other words, there is a single path for any current that flows through the circuit. When a circuit is wired in series, the total resistance of the circuit is the same as the sum of the resistances of all individual elements of the circuit. The total current of the circuit is equal to the current flowing through any given element at any time. The total voltage of the circuit is equal to the voltages across each element added together.

Parallel Circuit

Parallel circuits have elements that bridge the conductor. The circuit elements are not arranged linearly, as in a series circuit. This makes multiple paths for the current to flow through. In a parallel circuit, the total current is equal to the sum of the currents flowing across the circuit elements. The voltage of the circuit across any given circuit element is equal to the total voltage of the circuit, which means there is an equal voltage across each circuit element. To find the total resistance of a parallel circuit, the reciprocals resistances of each element are added together.

Imaging System

The power rating of an imaging system is typically given in kilowatts. Wattage is determined by multiplying the amperes (the measure of the current) by the voltage (the measure of electric potential). When working in milliamperes and kilovoltage peaks, the equation for the power rating is (mA x kVp)/1,000.

Using this equation, determine the power rating for an imaging system with the capability of producing 1,000 mA when operating with 120 kVp. The power rating would be (1,000 mA x 120 kVp)/1000, which is equal to 120 kW. Single-phase imaging systems are not as efficient. To determine the power rating of this kind of instrument, multiple the final answer by 0.7.

Secondary Voltage

A step-up transformer uses the principles of electromagnetic induction to increase the primary voltage from the power supply into a much higher voltage. This is necessary in an imaging system because very high voltages are needed to produce the electron flow within the x-ray tube. The transformer uses two coils of wire. The secondary coil has between 500 to 1,000 turns for every one turn of wire in the primary coil. When a current is introduced into the primary coil, it triggers a current in the secondary coil. The current can be found by multiplying the voltage peak in the primary coil by the turns ratio of the second coil. If a transformer has a turns ratio of 750 and a 120 Vp is used, then the secondary voltage peak will be 120 Vp x 750. That's 90,000 Vp or 90 kVp.

Important Terms

Matter: In physics, matter is anything that occupies physical space. Matter can take the form of a solid, liquid, or gas. Subatomic particles that possess mass would also be defined as matter.

Mass: Matter is measured by mass. In layman's terms, mass is treated as an equivalent to weight.

Energy: In physics, energy is defined as the ability of any amount of mass to do work.

Potential Energy: Depending on the position of a mass, there may be the possibility for it to release a certain amount of energy. For example, a ball held at a certain height has potential energy associated with its release and fall from that height.

Kinetic Energy: When a mass is set in motion, the resulting energy is referred to as kinetic energy.

Chemical Energy: Energy released during a chemical reaction.

Electrical Energy: When electrons move either in isolation or between molecules it creates electrical energy.

Thermal Energy: The movement of atoms and molecules releases heat, also known as thermal energy.

Nuclear Energy: A tremendous amount of energy is contained within the atomic nucleus. It is referred to as nuclear energy.

Electromagnetic Energy: Electromagnetic energy is generated within matter, and when emitted can transition through matter. Electromagnetic energy has a spectrum of energy levels. The energy level and the density of the matter exposed determine how much of the energy passes through it.

Atomic Nucleus: The central structure of an atom. Protons (positively charged subatomic particles) and neutrons (that do not carry a charge) are within the nucleus. The major part of an atom's mass is within the nucleus.

Atomic Mass: The atomic mass is equal to the number of neutrons and the number of protons contained within the nucleus.

Electron Shells: Electrons exist in an atom at specific distances from the nucleus. Their orbits are referred to as shells. They are identified by the letters K, L, M, N, O, P, and Q. A stable atom, meaning it does not carry an ion charge, has the same amount of electrons and protons.

Atomic Number of an Atom: The atomic number is based on the protons found in the nucleus. This is what determines the type of atom, as referenced to the elements found on the Periodic Table.

Isotopes: It is possible for the same type of atom, determined by the number of protons, to have differing numbers of neutrons. These are known as isotopes. For example, deuterium (heavy hydrogen) is an isotope of hydrogen.

Electron-binding Energy: A force exists within an atom that keeps the electrons in place and prevents them from collapsing into the positively charged nucleus. This is called the electron-binding energy.

Octet Rule: Electron shells never contain more than eight electrons at a time.

Particulate Radiation: This is made up of alpha and beta particles. Alpha particles consist of two protons and two neutrons without electrons. Beta particles are similar to electrons. They are released from radioactive atoms.

Photon: A particle of electromagnetic energy. Photons travel in a wave pattern at the speed of light. They have no mass. A photon may be also referred to as a quantum of electromagnetic energy.

Sine wave: The wave pattern that electromagnetic energy moves in. The height of the wave is called the amplitude; the distance between peaks is called the wavelength. A smaller wavelength means that the photons have more energy. This information is used to determine the spectrum of the electromagnetic energy in question.

Frequency: When electromagnetic waves are measured, the frequency refers to the number of sine wave peaks that pass the point of measurement during a set period of time.

Speed of Travel: All electromagnetic energy travels at the speed of light. The speed of light is 186,000 miles per second. Regardless of frequency, wavelength, or amplitude, this speed remains constant.

Gamma Rays: This specific frequency of electromagnetic energy is produced only by radioactive atoms. They are very energetic, and similar to x-rays, except for how they are generated.

Wave-Particle Duality: Electromagnetic energy exhibits behaviors of both particles and waves, depending on how the energy is being measured.

Attenuation: When an x-ray beam makes contact with matter, the energy transfers through the matter. Some is absorbed, resulting in a lower level of energy coming out of the object than entered it. This effect is called attenuation.

Laws of Conservation: The law of conservation of matter states that matter cannot be created or destroyed. The law of the conservation of energy states that energy cannot be created or destroyed.

Electrostatics: Also known as static electricity, this is the buildup of a stationary electrical charge.

Electrification: When a charge moves between two objects, it is called electrification.

Laws of Electrostatics: Equal charges repel each other, while differing charges attract each other. An electrostatic charge is on the surface of an object, concentrated at the point of the greatest curvature. Negative charges move to connect with positive charges. Positive charges remain stationary.

Methods of electrification: Static electricity is generated by friction and moves through contact or near contact of two differently charged objects.

Conductor: A conductor is a material that allows electrons to move freely through it. Examples of good conductors are: Copper; silver; gold; graphite; electrolyte solutions; and plasma.

Insulator: An insulator does not allow movement of electrons through it. Nonconductive insulators resist a charge and build heat. Insulators are poor conductors. Examples of insulators are: Plastic, glass, and ceramics.

Electric Current: Electric current is measured in amperes. It is the flow of electrons through a conductor or along a circuit.

Electromotive Force: The movement of electrons through a circuit has a force associated with it, which can vary. This electromotive force is measure in volts.

Electrodynamics: The study of electrons and their movement.

Semiconductor: Depending on the conditions, a semiconductor will act as either a conductor or an insulator. Semiconductors are used to make diodes and transistors for computers and radios. Examples of semiconductors are: Silicon, carbon, and germanium.

Electric Resistance: This is a measure of how difficult or easy it is for electrons to travel through a material.

Ohm's law: The voltage within a circuit will be equal to the current (measured in amperes) multiplied by the resistance. An Ohm is the unit of measurement for resistance.

Electric Circuits: A circuit is the path that electrons travel along.

Alternating Current (AC): In an alternating current, the electrons do not flow in the same direction all the time. Instead, they rapidly change direction back and forth, 50—60 times per minute. AC is household current. It is better for transmitting electricity over long distances than direct current, because the voltage can be modulated.

Direct Current (DC): In a direct current, the electrons travel in a single direction from a negative to a positive charge. Batteries generate DC.

Magnetic Field: When an electric charge is in motion, it generates a magnetic field. This magnetic field can convey magnetism to ferromagnetic objects, such as those made out of iron.

Magnetic poles: Magnetic fields have two poles, referred to as the north pole and south pole. The north pole of one magnet will attract the south pole of another, and repel the north pole of another magnet.

Laws of magnetics: Like poles repel each other and opposite poles attract. The amount of attractive or repellant force follows the inverse square law.

Solenoid: When conductive wire is formed into a stacked coil, the electron flow through the coiled circuit generates a magnetic field that is particularly strong within the center of the coil.

Electromagnet: A cylinder of iron within a solenoid. It concentrates the magnetic field generated by the solenoid.

Electromagnetic induction: When a conductor with a current passing through it comes in the vicinity of another conductor with no live current, its magnetic field can trigger a current in the second conductor.

Self-induction: Passing an alternating current through a conductor can create an opposing voltage within the same conductor.

Mutual Induction: The process of using one conductor to trigger a current flow in another conductor.

Electric Generator: A machine that converts mechanical energy into electric energy, usually an alternating current.

Single-phase, two-pulse alternating current: This is the simplest form of current. It travels in a sine wave, and pulses twice every wavelength, once at the top peak and once at the bottom peak.

Three-phase alternating current: A special wiring pattern creates waveforms that are 120 degrees out of phase, with either 6 or 12 pulses per wave cycle.

Electric Motor: A machine that generates mechanical power by using electrical power.

Transformer: A device that uses mutual induction to change the voltages of currents, either increasing or decreasing them.

Step-up Transformer: A primary coil is used to increase voltage in a secondary coil. Found in an x-ray circuitry to increase voltage into kilovoltage.

Step-down Transformer: Decreases voltage in the secondary coil and increases the current. Used in x-ray machines to increase the current reaching the cathode.

Autotransformer: Uses an electromagnet to make small increases to the voltage before the current enters the step-up transformer. Used to control the kVp setting.

Rectification: It is possible to change alternating current to direct current. The process is called rectification. The device is called a rectifier.

Line voltage compensation: An x-ray circuit requires constant power. Most power sources, such as those that power buildings, experience variation. The line voltage compensation makes sure the power used by the x-ray machine is constant.

Weight: The force of gravity works on all objects on the earth. Weight is the measure of this effect: The mass of the object X the acceleration created by the force of gravity.

Momentum: Momentum is often confused with the velocity of an object. It is actually a more specific measurement that multiplies the mass of an object by its velocity.

Work: In physics, work has a very specific meaning. It is the amount of force applied to an object over a distance.

Power: From work, it is possible to determine power. Power is the amount of work done over a specific period of time.

Heat: Molecules are in constant motion, which means they possess kinetic energy. The measure of the kinetic energy of molecules in motion is heat.

Medical Equipment Function-Operation

Beam Limitation

The collimator is a variable aperture device. It allows the radiographer to adjust the size of the opening that the x-ray beam passes through. Unlike a camera aperture, the collimator uses two sets of lead shutters to control the intensity of the beam. The two different shutters operate at right angles to each other. The first blocks radiation that is not properly focused. The second set restricts the beam. The cylinder cones are attached to the bottom of the collimator. They further limit the beam, blocking most, so that it exits from the machine in only a small circle. The aperture diaphragm is a piece of lead with a small opening in the middle. It is used for additional control over the size of the x-ray beam.

Beam Filtration

Filtration is another safety measure that reduces patient exposure to radiation during any single procedure. Specifically, the filters are designed to remove low-energy radiation that increases patient exposure, but does not help form a diagnostic image. There are two types of common filtration:

1. Inherent filtration occurs when the x-ray tube itself filters out some of the low-energy radiation, as does the insulating oil that is around the tube
2. Added filtration is achieved with aluminum sheets used near the window of the x-ray tube.

These two filtration types added together make up the total filtration of the machine. The filtration is not adjusted by the radiographer. It is calibrated by an expert annually and checked whenever there are suspected anomalies. If the radiographer believes the filtration is not working as it should, he or she should not use the machine in question until it has been checked by an expert.

Biometric Instruments

A biometric instrument is one that is meant to measure some aspect of the human body. A radiography instrument falls into this category. Biometric instruments generally fall into one or more of five different categories:

1. Information gathering: Some instruments are used strictly for gathering information in order to expand the knowledge possessed by the medical industry.
2. Diagnostic: Many instruments are designed to help identify anomalies or malfunctions within the physiology with the hope of being able to correct them. The x-ray machine falls primarily into the diagnostic category.
3. Evaluative: These machines help to determine proper function and that proper function is being maintained.

4. Monitoring: Instruments designed for this purpose help medical professionals to keep track of particular processes on an ongoing basis; they may monitor a hospitalized patient's heart rate, for example.

Most biometric instruments use a stimulus on a subject, usually a human patient. The stimulus is the signal directed at the subject with the aim of producing a particular result. In the case of the radiographic instrument, the stimulus is the x-rays. Biometric instruments use transducers to convert one type of signal into another. The x-rays are converted into an image when they are captured by the film. Biometric instruments have signal-conditioning equipment, which are the controls that allow the radiographer to adjust signal strength. Most biometric equipment includes display equipment and recording equipment. In the case of the x-ray machine, the film works as both of these components.

Control: In some circumstances, a patient may need a machine to control certain processes that are usually automatic, such as a respirator to control breathing.

Range: all the differing inputs at which the machine should operate and provide a reasonably accurate result.

Sensitivity: the minimum variation in input that will produce a different result that can be accurately measured.

Varying inputs produce alterations in the output. Those variations either progress in a linear manner along the instrument's range or in a non-linear manner. Linearity means that a change in the input anywhere within the range will produce the same amount of variation in the output.

Hysteresis: If the input of an instrument is adjusted during the measurement, it can introduce an error caused by approaching the desired input from a higher or lower level, which is called a hysteresis error.

Frequency Response: How results vary in sensitivity through the range of a measurement. A good frequency response will accurately reproduce the physiology being measured.

Accuracy: How free from error measurements the instrument is. Accuracy can be affected by the tolerances of electronic components, mechanical errors caused by movement of components within the instrument, temperature variations, or poor frequency response.

Signal-to-noise ratio: It is possible for background radiation to interfere with accuracy. A signal (i.e., beam) that is stronger than background radiation will produce better results.

Stability: The constancy of the instrument. An instrument that is able to quickly return to normal parameters after a disruption, such as a power surge, has greater stability than one that takes a long time to reach its normal state.

Simplicity: Human-introduced error is always a concern. Instruments with greater simplicity of operation help to reduce the potential for human error.

Measuring a Living System

Measuring any part of a living body presents six major difficulties:

1. It is inherently difficult to access any area within the body. The x-ray machine helps to overcome this difficulty by taking a picture using radiation that can pass through the body, depending on the density of tissues. However, the very nature of x-rays requires special precautions because of the damage they can cause to the body's tissues.
2. The data itself varies from subject to subject, which presents difficulties in recognizing that what is normal for one human body may not be normal for another.
3. There are many interrelationships within the systems of the human body that are not fully understood. Properly interpreting the data can be difficult because of lack of physiological knowledge.
4. It is not uncommon for electrical equipment to produce artifacts, which refers to extraneous information that is shown in the end-result. Artifacts can be caused by background radiation, electrical interference, or signal disruptions. The most common cause is patient movement.
5. Biometric instruments work by exposing the body to energy. A balance must be struck between using enough energy to produce a reliable result and low enough energy levels to ensure patient safety.
6. Safety considerations are always the primary concern, and they necessarily limit the radiographer's ability to take accurate biometric readings.

X-Ray Examination Rooms

There are many different types of imaging systems that can be found in an examination room. Despite the different shapes and sizes available, most examination rooms will have:

- An x-ray machine that uses a voltage range within 25 to 150 kilovolt peaks and a tube that generates currents within the 100 to1200 milliampere range
- At least one radiographic imaging instrument, usually attached to a movable crane (gantry), so that it can be adjusted over the top of the examination table
- A fluoroscopic imaging instrument, usually located beneath the examining table
- The examination table itself is usually made of a carbon fiber that will not interfere much with the radiation

Every x-ray instrument has an x-ray tube, a high-voltage generator, and an operating console. The operating console is usually located in an adjacent room to the examination room, with a viewing window that allows the radiographer to see the patient during the procedure. The operating console allows the radiographer to:

- Set the current and voltage within the x-ray tube to control the intensity and penetrability of the x-ray beam
- Control the line compensation and the exposure time

Modern day consoles are automated in many ways, but it is still important that the radiographer understand the functions and features of the machine.

Most x-ray imaging systems are designed to run on 220 V power. Some run on 110 V or 440 V. No matter the voltage that the machine requires, the AC line power of a building will not be consistent enough to run an x-ray machine and produce accurate, high-quality images. This is why imaging systems have line compensators. The line compensator uses a meter to measure the incoming power source. It then makes adjustments to keep the power input consistent and precise. The line compensator is wired to the autotransformer and makes automatic adjustments, so the radiographer does not need to monitor power supply while making measurements.

Kilovoltage Peak

The kilovoltage peak (kVp) controls the quality of the x-ray beam. Quality generally refers to the penetrability of the x-ray beam. The controls that allow the radiographer to adjust the kVp actually select connections along the autotransformer. The autotransformer receives steady voltage from the line compensator, and then it steps up the steady low voltage to a higher voltage, capable of triggering x-ray production within the instrument. The kVp settings allow the radiographer to control how much the voltage is stepped up, ultimately adjusting the quality of x-rays produced. The x-ray machine is equipped with a pre-reading voltmeter that allows the radiographer to check the kVp before exposing a patient to x-rays.

Milliamperes

A current passes from cathode to anode within the x-ray tube. The number of electrons that passes between the two per second is measured in milliamperes (mA). There is a filament within the instrument that emits the radiation. The rate at which electrons are released from the filament is determined by the temperature, which is measured in amperes (A). The whole process is controlled through a filament circuit. The voltage of the filament circuit is controlled by the autotransformers through a series of very precise resistors. The radiographer controls the level of current through the operating console. Typically, the current is static, but some instruments allow for the mA to be varied to reduce exposure time.

Timers

Different imaging systems use different timers to control the patient's length of exposure to radiation. The timer helps the radiographer to set the mA very specifically. The timer is responsible for completing and breaking the circuit that delivers current to the x-ray tube. There are five types of timers:

- Synchronous: A synchronous timer is unique to instruments with a synchronous motor. The motor works at exactly 60 revolutions per second. Synchronous timers work in multiples of 1/60 or one second.
- Electronic: An electronic timer is a sophisticated device and very accurate, capable of rapidly resetting for serial exposures. Electronic timers are the most common kind of timer.
- Mechanical: A mechanical timer is a simplistic timer that uses a spring to control the timing of the exposure. They are not very accurate and are most commonly found in portable and dental imaging systems.
- mA: A milliampere is a unit of current equal to one thousandth (10^{-3}) of an ampere. Multiplying the milliamperes of current within the x-ray tube by the time of exposure determines the number of x-rays emitted from the tube. This is equivalent to the optical density of the image, measured in milliamperes (mA). mA timers detect the product of mA, and the time, and stop the exposure when the right level of milliamperes has been reached.
- Automatic: The final type of timer is an automatic timer, called an automatic exposure control. This device determines when enough radiation has been emitted to produce the image and automatically breaks the circuit. This is the only type of exposure timer that does not require a radiographer to set it.

High-Voltage Generator and Voltage Rectification

An x-ray machine requires high voltage to function. It needs a kilovoltage current of a specific waveform in order to generate x-rays. The standard AC current that comes from the power company is much too low, so x-ray imaging systems need a high-voltage generator. The high-voltage generator includes a high-voltage transformer, a filament transformer, and rectifiers. The high-voltage transformer increases the voltage that it receives from volts into kilovolts. The rectifier changes the current from the standard power source from an alternating current (AC) into a direct current (DC). The generation of x-rays depends on electrons flowing from the cathode to the anode. If the electron current reversed, the heat could destroy the instrument. The rectifiers keep that from happening by transforming the current from alternating to direct.

Rectifiers

There are two different types of rectifiers used in Radiology:

- A vacuum tube rectifier uses a glass tube that has been emptied of air (evacuated). There is a filament, or coil or wire, at one end. When a current moves through this coil, it heats up. As it becomes heated, it releases electrons, which will travel from the heated coil through the tube toward a metallic plate at the opposite end of the tube. Vacuum tube rectifiers prevent a reverse current because the anode does not generate electrons; it only receives them from the cathode.

- A solid-state rectifier uses semiconductors to generate a current that will flow in only a single direction. It uses a combination of two types of semiconductors to create a junction called a solid-state diode.

An unrectified voltage has been stepped up from a low voltage to a higher voltage, but is still an alternating current (AC). This current looks like a sine wave, with positive and negative flow. During the positive flow, it travels through the x-ray tube as it should, but during the negative flow, the current disappears because the anode will not emit electrons. This creates an inverse voltage that can cause the x-ray tube to fail.

Half-wave rectification removes the negative flow but does not induce a positive flow during those moments when the current disappears because the anode will not emit electrons. The x-ray tube receives a pulsing current in this case, which uses power inefficiently and requires longer exposure time.

Full-wave rectification induces a positive flow during the original negative cycles. The flow still pulses, but at twice the rate of the half-wave rectified current.

External Components of the X-Ray Tube

The x-ray tube's external structure consists of three main parts: The support structure, the protective housing that surrounds the tube, and a glass or metal envelope. The x-ray tube and its protective components are weighty. They require significant support that also allows the x-ray tube to be moved and adjusted by the radiographer. Most imaging systems use a ceiling support system. Two sets of rails are mounted to the ceiling over the radiographic table. The sets of rails run perpendicular to each other to provide a complete range of movement for the x-ray machine. Some imaging systems use a column that runs from the floor to the ceiling. The x-ray can move up and down the column and the column can be moved around the room using rollers. A third support system is the C-Arm support. This has the greatest range of motion and is used for special procedures, like cardiovascular imaging.

X-rays travel in all directions with equal intensity, which is a problem for controlling the patient's exposure during imaging, and limiting the cumulative exposure of the staff to x-ray radiation as they work. To solve this problem, the x-ray tube is enclosed in a protective housing that allows radiation to leave primarily through a window, which is directed at the patient to produce the desired image. Any other radiation that escapes is called leakage radiation. A properly functioning protective housing limits leakage radiation to less than 100 mR/hr at a 1-meter distance. The protective housing also reduces the radiographer's risks of accidental electric shock.

The glass or metal envelope is the vacuum tube, in which two electrodes are encased. All the air is sucked from the tube (evacuated) to create a vacuum. One of the electrodes, called the cathode, can emit electrons that will flow to the other electrode, called the anode. Regardless of whether the tube is glass or metal, it must be designed to undergo enormous temperatures without compromising its integrity.

Glass tubes are typically made of Pyrex. Metal tubes are becoming more common because they last longer and produce more accurate results over their lifespan. In a glass tube, tungsten that vaporizes from the anode will collect on the inner surface of the tube and skew results. Metal envelopes prevent this problem.

X-Ray Tube Heat

An x-ray imaging system accelerates a high number of electrons from the cathode through the tube to the small target on the anode. The electrons that hit the target have a tremendous amount of kinetic energy. The energy within the imaging system can be controlled very exactly. When the electrons come into contact with the target, they excite the atoms within the target. Heat, electromagnetic energy, infrared light, and x-ray radiation are all produced. Only about 1% of the kinetic energy produced in the x-ray tube transforms into x-rays. Most of the rest becomes heat. The imaging system is inefficient, but it still produces very useful results.

Active and Passive Transducers

Active transducers convert nonelectrical inputs into an electrical signal. Magnetics, mechanics, chemical reactions, and pressure are examples of nonelectrical inputs that can be transformed into an electrical signal. Usually, with active transducers it is also possible to reverse the process and convert the electrical signal back into its nonelectrical form. While there are many possible ways to build an active transducer, only a limited number of those methods are practical in a clinical setting.

Passive transducers use a circuit to measure a physical variable. There is a direct current excitation and/or alternating current carrier signal that can be controlled as part of the circuit. As the function value of the circuit changes, it is possible to measure the physical variable. Passive transducers are always resistors, capacitors, or inductors.

Cathode, Filament, and Focusing Cup

Cathode: The negative component of the x-ray tube, the side that emits electrons when it becomes heated, is called the cathode. It is made up of the filament and the focusing cup.

Filament: The cathode has a small coil of wire about 1 or 2 centimeters long, coiled to about 2 millimeters in diameter. When heated, this filament emits electrons. A current of 4 amperes or more boils off the outer electrons. They separate from the filament. The filament is most commonly made of tungsten, which has high electron emissions.

Focusing Cup: The focusing cup houses the filament. The focusing cup carries a negative charge that helps to direct and focus the electron flow to the anode at the other end of the x-ray tube.

Filament Current and Dual-Focus Tube

Filament Current: A current runs through the filament. When the radiographer first starts the machine, the current is low to warm up the filament, a process that prevents sudden changes in current flow. When the patient is ready for imaging, the radiographer increases the filament current to the point where electrons are emitted. A small increase in the filament current leads to a very large increase in the x-ray tube current. The radiographer controls the filament current to control the current in the x-ray tube.

Dual-focus tube: Most x-ray imaging systems have two different focal points. One is small and used when precision or high spatial resolution is necessary to produce a useful result. The other is used when imaging larger body parts. To achieve this, two filaments are embedded within the focusing cup, one large and one small.

Anode, Target, and Rotating Anode

Anode: The positive side of the x-ray is called the anode. Imaging systems either use a stationary anode (common in dental imaging systems) or a rotating anode (common in general purpose imaging systems). The anode collects the electrons that come from the cathode and directs them back through the high-voltage generator. The anode helps the target to function properly, and it acts as a thermal radiator.

Target: The area of the anode that is meant to be hit by the electron flow is called the target. It is usually made of tungsten alloyed with another metal like rhenium, molybdenum, or rhodium.

Rotating Anode: When the anode is rotated, it makes a higher tube current possible. It provides a larger target, which helps to control heating. The faster the anode rotates, the higher the current within the tube. This makes shorter exposure times possible, which enhances patient safety.

Induction Motor and Line-Focus Principle

Induction Motor: The mechanism that turns a rotating anode. Inside the tube is a copper and iron shaft. Electromagnets spaced around the neck of the tube cause the inner shaft to rotate when a sequential electromagnetic charge passes through them. An induction motor can be put into reverse, which stops the anode from rotating very quickly.

Line-focus Principle: The target emits the x-ray beam through the focal spot. A smaller focal spot produces an image with better resolution. X-ray designs incorporating the line-focus principle angle the target to create a smaller effective focal spot. For example, a 10 mm X 1 mm focal line is shortened into a 1 mm X 1 mm square. Most diagnostic radiography uses a source-to-film distance of 1 m and an anode angle not less than 15. Microradiography uses a microfocus of 0.33 mm and an anode angle of 6.

Heel Effect: Reduced x-ray intensity and film density at the anode side of the field because of anode angling, or a worn, roughened anode surface.

Tungsten

Tungsten has three main qualities that make it effective as a target material:

- Atomic number: The atomic number of tungsten is 74. Its high atomic number means it is a massive element, which makes it efficient at producing x-rays, particularly high-energy x-rays.
- Thermal conductivity: Tungsten is very conductive. Its thermal conductivity is similar to that of copper, the best conductor. This means that it efficiently releases the heat that builds up in the x-ray generation process.
- High melting point: Because of the high-levels of heat produced when generating x-rays, it is imperative that the target material not melt during the process. The melting point of tungsten is 3,400° Celsius, making it possible for tungsten to withstand the heat of the x-ray process.

Optical Density

The optical density of an image is the amount of radiation that passed through the tissues to be captured by the film receptor. The blacker the area on the developed image is, the more dense the radiation exposure to that area of film. The resultant image is a reverse image (negative) of the tissues. The areas where the least radiation passes through, i.e. the bones show up whitest on the developed image. The optical density (or the blackness of an area of the film) is technically calculated as a ratio of the amount of light striking the developed image from the light box behind it, to the amount of light that is actually transmitted through the image.

Image Density

Image density is determined by the settings the radiographer uses to form the image: Milliampere setting; kilovoltage peak setting; the source-to-film distance; the film-screen combination; the grids; the beam restriction; the anatomy and pathology being imaged; the anode heel effect; and the filtration all affect the image density. The mA setting controls the current, which ultimately determines the amount of radiation emitted by the imaging system. The kVp affects the energy of the emitted x-rays. Higher kVp means higher energy, which results in greater density. The density falls inversely by the square of the distance that the x-rays have to travel before being captured by the film. The film-screen combination, the grids, the beam restriction, the anatomy, the heel effect, and the filtration each have a different effect on the quality of the final image, but none so great as the settings and the distance.

Contrast

The contrast is the appearance of differing densities in the image. Contrast is what makes it possible to view the details within the image. Images that are high contrast, featuring mostly blacks and whites, are called short-scale images. Low contrast images with many shades of gray are called long-scale images. The factors that influence contrast are: Kilovoltage peak; grids; beam restriction; filtration; and anatomy and pathology. The kVp setting affects the beam's energy, which in turn affects the absorption differential, and has a direct effect on contrast. Lower kVp settings mean higher contrast because the energy of the x-rays does not penetrate as much. Grids are used to reduce x-ray scattering when imaging a larger part of the anatomy. Lower scatter rates mean higher contrast. Beam restriction and filtration both help to focus the beam, which improves contrast. The density of the tissues being imaged has a large effect on penetration of the x-rays and, therefore, on the image contrast.

Recorded Detail

Recorded detail refers to image sharpness. Other terms that are synonymous include detail sharpness, definition, and image resolution. The detail of the final image is affected by: The distance between the object and receptor; the distance between the x-ray source and the receptor; the size of the focal spot; the film-screen combination; and patient movement. A short distance between the object being imaged and the film-screen produces more image detail. A longer distance between the image source and film-screen improves image detail. A small focal spot increases resolution. A slower film-speed combination improves resolution, but it also increases exposure time, so the radiographer must determine the proper balance. The radiographer instructs the patient to remain as still as possible to improve resolution.

Radiographic Film

Before 1914, x-rays were developed on glass plates. WWI made photographic glass scarce, so highly flammable cellulose nitrate was substituted. In 1924, cellulose triacetate was developed to avoid flammability. Since 1960, radiographic film is made of a thin polyester base tinted with blue dye, to improve contrast and cut glare. The base supports the emulsion, which is attached with adhesive, and covered with a protective layer. Unlike photographic film, radiographic film is seldom single-emulsion (coated on one side). Radiographic film is usually double-emulsion (two-sided coating), so it will not blur on intensifying screens. Emulsion is gelatin with 1.0—1.5 micron crystals of a silver halide suspended in it. Silver halide crystals have sensitivity specks of silver-iodo-bromide, which react to radiation exposure and hold images. Three important characteristics of film are its: Speed (how quickly it holds an exposure); contrast (faster film provides more contrast); and latitude (the range of exposures that will produce a useful image). Fast speed films have thick emulsion or a high concentration of silver halide crystals.

The film used for developing radiographic images, like any film, has specific handling and storage procedures. If the radiographer neglects the following procedures, the film could be damaged or destroyed.

Storage: Keep the film in a cool place. Temperatures should not exceed 68°F. Keep the humidity range between 40%—60%. Store the film on-end, in boxes that are out of the way of additional radiation exposure, fumes, or light.

Handling: Radiographic film is pressure-sensitive. Applying pressure to it can leave marks that will result in artifacts. Static can also damage the film. The radiographer must carefully discharge any static build-up on surfaces the film will contact. Handle film gently. Do not bend or scratch film.

Intensifying Screens

An intensifying screen helps direct the exposure to the film and makes the film speed faster. The intensifying screen has a backing made of polyester and a reflective layer that directs the light toward the film, which is how it increases the speed. The active layer, called the phosphor layer, is fused to the base. It contains phosphorous crystals that emit visible light when in contact with radiation. Finally, a protective layer over the active layer protects the screen from scratches or other damage. The speed of the intensifying layer depends on the type of phosphor used, how large the crystals are, the thickness of the active layer, and how efficiently it reflects light.

Imaging System

Some imaging systems use strips of lead situated between aluminum spacers to form a grid that reduces the scatter radiation produced during imaging procedures. The scattered radiation travels in paths different from the imaging beam, and is usually absorbed by the grid. This absorption reduces ambient exposure to the radiographer and the patient. The ratio between the height of the lead strips and the space between them is the grid ratio. It is usually between 4:1 and 16:1. The grid frequency refers to the number of strips per inch, which ranges between 60—150. There are three primary types of grids: Linear, focused, and crossed grids. In a linear grid, the strips are parallel to each other. In a focused grid, the strips are situated at an angle that is best suited to absorb divergent radiation. In a crossed grid, there are two parallel grids set perpendicular to each other.

Grid Characteristics and Common Motion

The primary characteristics of a grid are:

- Enhancement of the resulting images: The improvement of contrast is described as a ratio between the contrast with the grid and without the grid. Some grids are stationary, and the resulting images may show grid lines. Other grids move back and forth during the procedure, to prevents visible grid lines.
- Scatter radiation absorbency: Selectivity is the measure of how efficiently the grid gathers scatter radiation. It is described as the ratio of the primary radiation to the secondary radiation. A higher selectivity ratio indicates better efficiency.
- Grid conversion factor: The grid conversion factor describes how much of an increase in exposure is required when using the grid. As the grid absorbs scatter radiation, it also affects the primary radiation used for imaging. The radiographer increases the mA setting to compensate for this absorption, which is also referred to as the Bucky factor.

Air Gap Technique

The air gap technique uses an increased object-to-image distance to help control scatter during certain procedures. The increased object-to-image distance means that scatter radiation will pass through the patient at divergent angles and miss the film. In some cases, such as taking an image of the lateral cervical spine, an increased object-to-image distance is unavoidable. In these cases, the extra distance simulates the effects of a grid and using a grid would only increase the exposure time to which the patient is subjected. In procedures such as a cerebral angiography, the distance is used in conjunction with a grid to keep exposure times to a minimum.

Technique Chart

Because the radiographer performs so many different radiographic procedures, it is difficult to remember optimum settings and techniques for everyone. The problem is further compounded by the variety of differences in patient size and shape (habitus). The technique chart can help. Use calipers to measure the thickness of the area to be imaged. Consult fixed kVp-variable mA or variable kVp technique charts. Use a kVp-variable mA chart first, because kVp doesn't change unless the part to be measured is unusually thick. The chart recommends the optimum settings, based on the thickness of the area. Thick areas require more radiation than thin areas. If the patient has unusual pathology, is very old or young, or has difficulty remaining still, the radiographer must make appropriate variations.

Chemicals

The developer is used to produce a visible image from the exposed silver bromide crystals. It uses reducing agents like hydroquinone and phenidone to build blacks and grays within the image. It uses an activator, like sodium carbonate, to soften the emulsion. Glutaraldehyde is used to control the sodium carbonate reaction, so that the film can pass through the processors undamaged. A restrainer, such as potassium bromide, prevents the reducing agents from developing unexposed silver bromide crystals. A preservative, like sodium sulfite, keeps the reducing agents from oxidizing. To finish the developing process, water is used to wash away the chemicals.

Once an image has been developed, it has to be fixed so that the developing chemicals don't over-develop the image. The fixer contains a fixing agent, also known as hypo. Most often this is ammonium thiosulfate. It works to shed the remaining, unexposed crystals of silver bromide. The fixer also contains an acidifier, composed of acetic acid. It works to neutralize the alkaline developer solution. It also contains a hardener, usually aluminum chloride. This reacts with the emulsion, causing it to shrink and harden. Hardening prepares the film for viewing and storage. Like the developer, the fixer contains sodium sulfite as a preservative that slows the rate of oxidation when the fixer is exposed to air. Finally, water is used as a solvent to dissolve and remove the chemicals after the process is complete.

AUTOMATIC PROCESSING

Most radiographic images are developed using an automatic processor. It controls the developer and fixer mix, so that the chemicals are properly balanced. It also controls the amount of time that the images spend in each stage of the development process. An automatic processing machine uses a transport system to move the film through the development process at the proper pace. It uses rollers that catch and move the film. The entrance roller grabs the film and transports in into the developer tank. After development is complete, larger rollers catch the image and move it through the fixer and wash tanks and then into the drying section. The final step is a squeegee assembly that removes the bulk of the remaining water.

The automatic processing machine replenishes the developer solution and the fixer solution every time an image is developed. The initial rollers catch the film and pull it into the processing machine, which triggers the release of fresh solutions into their respective tanks. There are holding tanks for the fresh solution that are connected to the automatic processor by tubes. During replenishment, the solutions move from the holding tanks into the system. To prevent too much solution from being fed into the system, the radiographer should feed the film into the system along its short aspect. Keep the temperature of the developer and fixer solutions as constant as possible. Agitating and recirculating the solutions helps to achieve this. It also puts the solutions through a filtration system, which helps to remove particles that have been introduced by the development process.

By properly caring for the automatic processing system, the radiographer can prevent image distortions from being introduced by the development process and can extend the life of the machine:

Start-up Procedure	Shut-down Procedure
Every time you turn the machine on: 1. Close the wash tank valve 2. Activate the water source 3. Turn on the processor 4. Wash the crossover racks where the film is moved between tanks 5. Replace the lid 6. Run several films through the processor 7. Check the replenishment rates and the temperature of the developer	Every time you shut off the machine: 1. Turn off the water first 2. Turn off the processor 3. Open up the wash tank valve 4. Allow the tank to drain 5. Wash the crossover racks again 6. Do not close the machine's lid all the way after shut-down — leave it slightly open to prevent condensation, which can dilute or alter the developer solution

Digital Fluoroscopy

Digital fluoroscopy transfers the image directly to a computer for analysis. It does not require development of the film by using solutions and a processing machine. Instead, an analog signal travels through an analog-to-digital converter. This device takes the information about contrast and image detail and converts into numerical data. The numerical data is then converted into an image that can be viewed on a high-resolution monitor. Another advantage of digital fluoroscopy, besides not needing development solutions, is that the image can be manipulated without destroying the original information. Digital fluoroscopy uses an imaging plate made of photostimulable phosphor. Accurate positioning and proper procedure are still necessary to get a useful image.

A digital fluoroscopy image has a wider exposure latitude than conventional imaging systems. This means that the radiographer can capture useful images at a wider range of exposures. Usually, the digital image is also better than a film image, and is easier to read. Because the image is digital, the radiographer can improve the image without altering the original information. Information not of interest can be removed. The edges and the contrast can be enhanced. The image can even be reversed, making the densest areas black and the least exposed areas white.

Characteristic Radiation

X-rays are actually produced by projectile electrons, fast-moving electrons that collide with the heavy-metal atoms within the target. When one of the electrons hits a target atom with enough energy to disrupt inner shell electrons, a reaction takes place that produces x-rays. Usually, it is electrons in the outer shell that are knocked off. When an inner-shell electron is knocked out, it puts the atom into a severely unnatural and imbalanced state. An outer-shell electron will quickly collapse into the hole created by the missing inner electron. When it does, an x-ray is produced. X-ray energy is equivalent to the energy that bound the involved electrons into their orbits, and is known as characteristic radiation.

Bremsstrahlung X-Rays

When an inner-shell electron is knocked out of place and an outer-shell electron replaces it, a very specific amount of energy is produced. Only the x-rays produced from a K-shell electron being knocked are energetic enough to be useful diagnostically. (Other shells further out from the nucleus produce lower energy x-rays when affected, and do not produce good images.) In addition to the characteristic radiation, some electrons pass near enough to the nucleus to have their kinetic energy affected by its surrounding field. The field forces the electrons to slow down, and an x-ray with energy corresponding to that lost by the electrons is emitted. This is bremsstrahlung radiation. It exists in a much wider range than characteristic radiation. Bremsstrahlung radiation makes up the bulk of the diagnostic beam.

Information on Developed Images

In addition to the image itself, these identifying markers should appear on each image you develop, enabling you to keep good, organized records, making subsequent diagnostics of the same area easier, and more likely to be accurate:

- Patient's full name
- Unique identifier, such as a medical record number
- Date of birth
- Date the image was made, so that age comparisons can be made over time
- Anatomic markers, such as right and left, top and bottom, made with a radiopaque marker
- Time interval, if a specific time interval was used to make the image
- Patient's orientation (standing up or lying down, for example)
- Whether the image was taking during inspiration or expiration, if the image is of the chest
- Sequence markers, if the image is part of a series

X-Ray Emission Spectra

X-rays emitted from the imaging system have a variety of different energies and wavelengths. The amount of different x-ray energy emissions is determined by the energy of the electrons striking the target. Many of them will have low energies and some will have high energies. The energies of the electrons going into the target affect the energy of the x-rays that will be released. The thickness of the target can also affect the x-ray emissions. Bremsstrahlung x-rays that result from multiple interactions of projectile electrons will have lower energy. Often, the target itself will absorb low-energy electrons, which decreases the number of low-energy electrons in the emitted beam. Filtration also removes some of the low-energy electrons from the beam.

The milliampere setting affects the number of electrons that flow between the cathode and the anode. It is a linear relationship. If the radiographer doubles the mA setting, the number of electrons in flowing through the x-ray tube will also double. The mA setting does not alter the energy levels of the x-rays emitted from the tube, but it does increase the number of x-rays emitted.

When the kilovoltage peak (kVp) setting is increased, it also increases: The number of electrons flowing through the tube; the number of x-rays emitted; and the average energy of the x-rays being emitted. The kVp setting determines the maximum energy that the x-rays can have.

Filtration devices are meant to absorb low-energy x-rays, while allowing diagnostically useful, higher energy x-rays to pass through the object being imaged. A filtration device changes the spectra of the emitted beam by reducing the number of x-rays that pass through, while increasing the average energy of those x-rays.

The target material will change both the quality and quantity of the x-rays in the emitted beam. Materials with a higher atomic number provide more characteristic radiation from the K-shells of the atoms. In other words, heavier target materials produce higher energy x-rays. The type of voltage waveform produced by the x-ray generator will affect the both the quantity and the energy of the result x-rays. The rectification used affects the number of electrons in the overflow, which in turn affects the number of x-rays emitted.

Medical Equipment Problem Solving

Standard Safety Procedures

X-ray radiographers are required to recognize the dangers of radiation to their patients and to take measures to reduce and control the exposure that their patients receive. These same precautions will also help to extend the life of the system. The primary source of wear and tear, and the usual cause of eventual breakdown, comes from using higher mA or kVp settings than necessary and using longer exposure times. By keeping the mA and kVp settings as low as possible, the radiographer can reduce the stress on the imaging system. Lowering exposure times and using faster image receptors can extend the life of the system. Avoiding repeat exposures will also reduce wear and tear. By practicing good safety habits, the radiographer will also help to prolong the useful life of the imaging system.

Image Distortion

Distortion occurs whenever there is an artifact produced by the image receptor that changes the size or shape of the anatomic structure being imaged. In other words, a distortion produces an inaccuracy in the results. The two types of distortion are in size and shape.

- Distortions in size occur from magnifying the image, from positioning the object and the image receptor too far apart, or from using too short a distance between the x-ray source and the image receptor. In these cases, the anatomy in question appears to be larger than it is.
- Distortions in shape happen when an image becomes elongated or conversely shortened. Both types of shape distortion happen when the imaging system or part of the imaging system is not properly aligned.

Heat Dissipation

The most common cause of early x-ray failure is over-heating within the unit. The imaging system generates a great deal of heat. If it does not dissipate properly, then the x-ray tube is damaged and loses function. The three ways that heat dissipates are through radiation, conduction, and convection. Radiation is when the heat is released through infrared radiation. Conduction is when heat moves through an object. Convection is when heat is released during an object's movement. The x-ray machine depends on all methods of dissipation. The heated anode releases infrared radiation. Heat from the anode conducts down the neck and moves into the glass envelope. As the glass envelope heats up, it also heats the surrounding oil bath. Convection occurs within the bath, which moves heat to the housing, where it is released into the air.

Excessive Heat

If the anode reaches a temperature that is too high, parts of the anode may begin to melt. This will cause pitting on the anode's surface. When the surface becomes pitted, the radiation emissions from the system are affected. The output may become less predictable and generally lower. If a high degree of melting occurs, some of the tungsten will begin to vaporize and coat the inside of the envelope—a particular problem if the envelope is made of glass. The tungsten coating can disrupt the electron flow within the tube.

If the anode is brought to a high temperature too quickly, it may crack or begin rotating unstably. Either situation will cause the x-ray tube to fail. The anode should always be warmed up before using, inducing maximal radiation for a procedure.

When the anode is heated for a procedure, the intense temperatures usually last between 1—3 seconds. The heat is dissipated through radiation, conduction, and convection. The heat that is conducted through the neck of the tube causes the rotor assembly to heat up. This can affect the bearings, causing imbalance during anode rotation. Damage to the bearings is another common reason that imaging systems fail. Bearing failure is usually more of risk during fluoroscopy. While the procedure does not require as much heat as radiography, the heat is usually prolonged, which is more likely to overheat and damage the bearings.

X-Ray Tube Failure

Excessive heating not only damages the anode; it can also affect the filament in the cathode. If the filament wire, which is made of tungsten, overheats, the tungsten begins to vaporize. The vaporized tungsten from both the cathode and the anode coats the inside of the envelope. On occasion, the build-up of tungsten on the inside of the envelope will interfere with the electron flow. In the worst cases, the interference can cause the tube current to arc, which causes failure. Tungsten vaporization also causes the filament wire to thin. If it becomes too thin, it will break, causing the filament to burn out. Proper use extends the life of the machine. Most correctly used imaging systems will process at least 50,000 exposures before the tube is at risk for failure.

Grid Errors

The radiographer can introduce errors into the x-ray image by installing the grid upside down, off-level, or off-center. Installing the grid upside down causes optical density to fade at the edges of the image. Install focused grids so that the labeled side faces the x-ray tube. When a grid is off-level, optical density will decrease across the entire image. To prevent this, ensure that the grid is perpendicular to the center ray. An off-center linear grid results in lateral decentering. The central ray does not strike the grid in the proper place. A focused grid that is off-center results in grid-focus decentering, which causes lower optical density at the sides of the image.

Image Artifacts

The imaging instrument is not the only place in which problems can occur. The processor can also malfunction and introduce errors. Artifacts are marks or divergent exposures that occur on the film and give either false information or confuse the accurate information that is present. One cause of artifacts is scratches from the guide shoes. The guide shoes are the part of the processor that grab and guide the film through the developing process. They can leave scratches in straight lines on the film. These lines will appear at evenly spaced intervals and will run in the same direction as the film travels. Adjusting the guide shoes into proper alignment can eliminate this problem.

Pi lines are another cause of image artifacts. These are small marks on the film after processing. When they are caused by one-inch rollers, the marks appear 3.141 inches apart; hence, they are called pi marks. A damaged roller causes these marks. A small nick on the roller leaves a small scratch on the film every time that part of the roller comes in contact with the film. Chemical stains, dirt, or debris on the roller can cause a similar effect. To correct this problem, the radiographer must either clean or replace the roller. Take care during cleaning to prevent further nicks to the roller.

Temperature fluctuations in the developer solution can cause artifacts. When the developer becomes hotter than it should be, it could result in optical densities that are too high, or that are foggy. When the developer temperature is too low, the density levels of the resulting image are lower than they should be. In both cases, the radiographer must adjust the thermostat that regulates the developer temperature to correct the problems.

Improper temperatures in the dryer stage can leave the film more susceptible to damage. When the film comes out of the processor, it should be dry to prevent scratches during handling. If the film is damp when it comes out, the radiographer needs to increase the dryer temperature. When ambient humidity is high, the radiographer increases the dryer temperature to compensate. To reduce humidity, the radiographer can also remove the front of the processor for a short time, to allow some of the humidity to dissipate out of the machine.

Scatter Radiation

Scatter radiation results from x-rays that interact with atoms in such a way that their path is changed. These x-rays don't reach the image receptor. Higher levels of scatter radiation reduce image quality by lowering the contrast of the image, and by causing the image to blur. The three main things that affect the scatter radiation are: The kVp level; the field size; and the thickness of the area to be x-rayed. The radiographer has control over the kVp setting and the field size, but not the thickness of the patient's anatomy. Adjusting the kVp level may seem like an easy solution, but often lowering kVp requires an increase in mA levels to get the needed image. The end-result is a higher x-ray dosage for the patient. Adjusting field size is a practical way to cut radiation. Smaller field sizes (the breadth of the image) make for less scatter radiation. Adjusting aperture, using cones and cylinders to control the beam, and using grids can all help to lower scatter radiation.

Geometric Factors

Geometric factors are those that are determined by positioning and the angle of the x-rays reaching the receptor. The three main geometric factors that can affect image quality are magnification, distortion, and focal-spot blur. Whenever a radiographic image is captured, some degree of magnification occurs. That means the image is larger than the actual size of the object imaged. Smaller levels of magnification result in higher quality images. In most images, there is a degree of unevenness of magnification that is caused by positioning. This results in image distortion. The radiographer can reduce distortion by paying careful attention to positioning, but not all distortion is avoidable. Focal-spot blur results from a large effective focal spot (most imaging systems have a focal spot that is rectangular and up to 1.5 mm on a side). When a large focal spot is combined with a short source-to-image distance and a long object-to-image receptor distance, focal-spot blurring will occur.

Image Distortion

Image distortion occurs when magnification is uneven across the object being imaged. The factors that can cause image distortion are: The thickness of the object being imaged; the positioning of the object; and the shape of the object. Most body parts that the radiographer images vary in thickness, which changes the distance between the object and the image receptor from one point to the next (OID). A varying OID results in some distortion. The object to be imaged must be positioned at the central axis of the x-ray beam, or unequal magnification will result, causing distortion. Finally, the shape of the object may cause unevenness in the magnification levels across the image.

Focal-Spot Blur

To calculate the area affected by focal spot blur, you must know the area of the effective focal spot, the distance between the x-ray source and the object to be imaged (SOD), and the distance between the object to be imaged and the image receptor (OID). The equation used is focal-spot blur (FSB) = (effective focal spot) (OID/SOD). Example: If an x-ray tube has an effective focal spot of 0.5mm, and it is used to take an image of an object within the abdominal cavity that is estimated to be 5 cm from the anterior wall of the abdomen, determine the focal-spot blur if the SOD is 160 cm and the image receptor is 6 cm from the tabletop.

$$\text{FSB} = 0.5\text{ mm} \times ((5+6)\text{cm}/(160-5-6)\text{cm})$$
$$\text{FSB} = 0.5\text{ mm} \times 0.073$$
$$\text{FSB} = 0.0369\text{ mm}$$

Ensuring Useful, High Quality Images

The radiographer ensures the production of a high-quality image through these steps:

- Take time to discuss the procedure with the patient. Communicate the importance of stillness and proper position of the area to be imaged.
- Choose the right type of imaging device and the proper film-screen combination for the given circumstances.

- Select the proper technique that will best suit the imaging requirements. This means deciding on the kVp, mA, and time exposure settings that will minimize the patient's exposure, while capturing a useful, high quality image on the first try.

To obtain the best possible image on the first attempt, determine the proper technique:

1. The radiographer's first step is to assess the patient's body type, or habitus. The typical body habitus is sthenic; this patient is strong and of average build. Patients who are thinner than average, but still healthy, are called hyposthenic. Overweight or massively-built patients are hypersthenic. Patients who are frail are asthenic. Technique charts use sthenic as a baseline. The radiographer must know what adjustments to make for the four body habitus types.
2. After body habitus, the radiographer measures the thickness of the body part with calipers, and selects the proper technique.
3. After thickness, the radiographer assesses body composition, and the composition of the area to be imaged, which have significant effects on the technique to be used.
4. Finally, the patient's pathology affects the technique.

Fixed and High kVp Charts

While there are a variety of charts available to the radiographer, the two most frequently used are the fixed kVp chart and the high kVp chart. When using a fixed kVp chart, the radiographer selects the kVp to be used for the examination based on the anatomy. Once the kVp is selected, the radiographer adjusts the mA and exposure time, based on body habitus type, thickness, and composition. The high kVp chart works in the same manner as the fixed kVp chart, but it is used for special circumstances that require kVp values over 100. The high kVp chart is used in x-rays of the chest cavity and in those using barium as a contrast medium.

Tomography

Taking an x-ray image of the chest or abdomen cavity is difficult. There are many soft-tissue structures that are exposed, and in the developed image they are superimposed on each other. The “stacked” tissues make chest and abdominal images difficult to read. The specific structure the radiologist needs to examine may not be clear enough to make a useful diagnosis. In these situations, doctors order tomography, a technique that improves the contrast resolution of the image. In tomography, the image receptor and the x-ray tube move together. Tomographic technique helps increase the contrast resolution, to make the structure of interest more visible. Tomography is also called body section radiography, planigraphy, laminography or stratigraphy, because the object detail from only one plane or region is sharply focused.

The most common form of tomography is linear tomography, in which the x-ray tube and the image receptor move in a synchronized and linear fashion. Linear tomography is most often used to identify calcified kidney stones (uroliths) and to take images of the cervical spine, thoracic spine, lumbar spine, chest, intravenous pyelogram (IVP), and wrist. Tomography was used more frequently in the past, when circular, elliptical, hypocycloidal, and trispiral tomography first made high contrast images of many anatomical structures feasible. Circular tomography is useful for cardiac imaging. Elliptical tomography is useful for the middle ear, sternum, and myocardium. Hypocycloidal tomography is useful for viewing the bony orbit of the eye, ear ossicles, and for measuring the mandible before implants are inserted in the jaw. Trispiral tomography is particularly useful for staging Kienböck's disease, palatal defects in children, and scaphoid fractures. However, computed tomography (CT) and magnetic resonance imaging (MRI) have largely replaced the use of tomography for most procedures.

Stereoradiography

Stereoradiography makes radiographical images appear three-dimensional. The radiographer makes two images of the same object. A stereoscope allows the viewer to look at one image with one eye and the other image of the same object with the other eye. The overall effect of viewing an image like this is that the object appears three-dimensional. Stereoradiography is another practice that is becoming outdated. Sophisticated computer programs can now make CT and MRI results into a three-dimensional image. This latter method of constructing a three-dimensional image is now mainstream.

Magnification Radiography

In some fields of medicine, the structures are small enough that magnification is needed to be able to observe the object of interest in any sort of useful way. While magnification is usually something the radiograph tries to limit, when small blood vessels must be examined, magnification is actually desirable. Magnification radiography is usually performed by vascular radiologists and neuroradiologists. The object-to-image receptor distance is increased, while the source-to-image distance remains the same. The overall effect is a magnified image that makes it possible to view very small structures.

Conventional radiography images areas with varied composition, so it is fairly noise-free. Fat, muscles, organs, and bones all have different densities, so the imaging technique is straightforward. Soft tissues are invisible or very low-contrast in conventional radiography, but are the most likely tissues to develop disease processes. A breast mammogram is the most common soft-tissue image.

Deformed soft tissues are problematic for the radiographer and surgeon. To make noise-free diagnostic images of soft tissues, the radiographer changes the target composition, the size of the focal spot, and the type of filtration. The radiographer may need to use acoustic resonance imaging or water-filled phantoms for soft tissues. When a CT scanner is unavailable, the radiographer requires a flat panel C-arm fluoroscopic unit for soft tissue imaging. Soft tissue deformities make it difficult for the surgeon to perform image-guided surgery. The surgeon must landmark with nearby bony structures, particularly for cardiac and orthognathic surgery (where an oral and maxillofacial surgeon repairs a cleft palate or craniofacial deformity).

Mammogram Imaging Systems

For most imaging systems, the target is made of tungsten. For mammogram imaging systems, the target is made specifically from tungsten alloyed with molybdenum or rhodium. A tungsten target produces a great deal of energy from bremsstrahlung x-rays, which is absorbed by the patient, but does not help to produce a useful diagnostic image. By including molybdenum with tungsten in the target, the x-ray spectrum shifts and includes more energy in the useful range, and excludes much of the bremsstrahlung radiation. A target made with rhodium will have a similar shift in spectrum, but will have more bremsstrahlung radiation than that of the molybdenum/tungsten target.

The focal-spot size of a mammographic x-ray tube must be much smaller than that of a conventional imaging system. Mammographic imaging requires the ability to capture images of very small calcifications within the soft breast tissue. Mammographic focal spots are often sized down to 0.1 millimeter. Smaller focal spots are better; however, shape also affects the imaging ability of the system. The ideal focal-spot shape is a circle. Manufacturers are able to design the x-ray tube in such a way that small rectangular focal spots can also be effective. With such a small focal spot, producing x-rays at a high enough intensity is difficult. Manufacturers use angling techniques to make the effective focal spot smaller, while still allowing adequate radiation through for imaging.

Because the mammographic imaging system is designed to take images of soft tissue, special filtration requirements must be taken into account. The window of the mammographic x-ray tube is usually made of either beryllium or borosilicate glass. In addition to the filtration that is provided by the window, a molybdenum or rhodium filter is also used. This is meant to bring the total filtration up to the equivalent of 0.5 mm of aluminum. This is the bare minimum of filtration required in a mammographic imaging system. The ideal filter may change, depending on the characteristics of the patient's breasts.

In mammography, the heel effect (where the intensity of the beam is reduced when the x-ray tube is angled) is used advantageously. Because of the uneven shape of the breast — it is thicker adjacent to the chest — adjustments must be made in order to capture an even exposure. If the cathode end of the x-ray tube is positioned closer to the chest wall and coupled with a long source-to-image distance of 60—80 centimeters, then it is possible to even out the exposure. The mammographer uses compression to compensate for the difference in tissue thickness across the breast.

Mammography uses a smaller focal point, an alloyed target, special filtration considerations, and the heel effect to overcome the unique challenges presented in imaging breast tissue. In addition to these adjustments, the mammographer places the patient's breast between two metal plates and compresses it to a more even thickness. This makes a uniform exposure more attainable. The compressed breast is also closer to the image receptor, and this reduces focal-spot blur (FSB). In addition, compression reduces scatter radiation and holds the breast still, which reduces blur. The overall effect of breast compression is better image quality and less radiation exposure for the patient.

The lower kVp settings for mammograms increase the image contrast, but not enough to make the imaging as reliable as needed. Grids are used in nearly every mammography system in order to increase contrast. Usually, the grids have a 4:1 or 5:1 ratio. Grid frequencies in mammography systems of 30—50 lines per centimeter are common. Some mammography systems use a special kind of grid, called a high transmission cellular grid (HTC grid), which reduces scatter radiation in two directions. Automatic exposure control devices are also routinely used. They are placed behind the image receptor and measure both the x-ray intensity and the x-ray quality to help ensure that an adequate image is captured without overexposure. The two types of automatic exposure control devices used in mammography systems are usually ionization chambers or solid-state diodes.

Mammography presents unique challenges for image contrast. Originally, four different types of image receptor played a role in increasing contrast: Direct-exposure film, xeroradiography, film-screen, and digital detectors. Only film-screen and digital detectors are used currently. Film-screen combinations that are designed specifically for mammography use a single-emulsion and single-back screen to cut light crossover. The emulsion used in mammographic image receptors is different than those used in standard receptors. Mammography uses a cubic grain, rather than a tabular grain, to further increase contrast. An intensifying screen speeds image capture and reduces patient exposure. The film-screen combination is positioned in the imaging system in a cassette made especially for mammography. Film-screen captures have better spatial resolution than digital detectors, but digital is gaining popularity because the image can be manipulated easily with computer software.

The charged couple device (CCD) is a type of image receptor. It is a solid-state device that can charge visible light photons into electrons to make greater spatial resolution possible. Spatial resolution is one of the shortcomings of digital mammography. Even with a CCD, the spatial resolution is still not as good as film-screen captures. The advantages to digital mammography are higher contrast and the availability of post-processing technology — the image can be adjusted using computer software programs. Not all digital mammography uses a CCD at this point. Some use thin-film transistors of image capture. Most still use thallium-activated cesium iodide. While digital mammography is still limited by spatial resolutions, as the technology improves, it is conceivable that digital will become the standard.

Mammography Quality Standards Act

The Mammography Quality Standards Act lays out specific roles for the radiologist, the medical physicist, and the mammographer to ensure:

- Patient safety
- The best possible image is produced
- The patient receives appropriate care during the procedure

The radiologist is considered the supervisor, and is responsible for implementing and overseeing a quality-control program, as part of a broader goal of quality assurance. The radiologist is also responsible for maintaining open lines of communication with the patient. The radiologist ensures that procedures are in place for communicating with patients both during a procedure and after a procedure, should follow-up be needed. The radiologist should encourage everyone in the office to always be thinking of ways to further improve the quality of care delivered to the patient.

The Mammography Quality Standards Act lays out specific roles for the radiologist, the medical physicist, and the mammographer to ensure patient safety, to ensure that the best possible image is produced, and to ensure that the patient receives appropriate care during the procedure. The primary responsibility of the medical physicist is to ensure that the mammography equipment is functioning within its specifications. The medical physicist must evaluate each piece of equipment annually, and whenever a component has been replaced or repaired. The medical physicist often plays the role of problem-solver, and must be familiar with the imaging process to do so. The medical physicist works closely with the mammographer to help the mammographer predict and overcome imaging problems.

The Mammography Quality Standards Act lays out specific roles for the radiologist, the medical physicist, and the mammographer to ensure patient safety, to ensure that the best possible image is produced, and to ensure that the patient receives appropriate care during the procedure. The mammographer has the most direct interaction with the patient during the mammography procedure. The mammographer is responsible for the daily commission of the quality control program. If there are several mammographers in the same office, then one mammographer should lead the quality control program. To ensure the quality of care given to each patient, the mammographer is expected to carry out 12 tasks, some of them daily, some weekly, and some less frequently.

Mammographer Quality Control Tasks

To ensure quality control, the mammographer has 12 tasks to perform at regular intervals. Two of these tasks must be performed on a daily basis:

Maintain a clean environment in the darkroom. During development, anomalies can be introduced into the image, which compromises image quality. A clean darkroom is the first step to reducing darkroom errors. The quality control mammographer ensures the:

- Darkroom's floor is mopped each day
- Counters are cleared of all items and wiped down
- Processor feed tray on the developer machine is cleaned

The quality control mammographer checks the processor every day to ensure it:

- Is in working order
- Has been calibrated
- Has correct mid-density levels, density difference, and base plus fog levels

The quality control mammographer must ensure that a new or newly repaired processor is working properly to reduce artifacts in the developed images. The mammographer:

1. Checks that the chemical system is working as it should
2. Cleans the tanks and racks
3. Adds developer replenisher, fixer, and developer starter fluids to the proper tanks in the amount specified by the manufacturer
4. Measures the temperature of the developer (not with a mercury thermometer)
5. Turns on the processor and allows the instrument to warm up
6. Measures the optical densities of the mid-density step, the density difference, and the base plus fog using a sheet of film and sensitometer
7. Records the results in a log to establish baseline values
8. Compares daily measurements with the baseline to confirm that the instrument is functioning properly

Weekly tasks:

1. Clean the screens used in image capture. When dirt or dust accumulates on intensifying screens, the image may appear to have microcalcifications that are not really there. This can lead the radiologist to a wrong diagnosis. The screens should be cleaned each week according to manufacturer instructions. Also, if any dust or dirt is noticed on a screen, it should be cleaned immediately, rather than waiting for the weekly cleaning.
2. Clean the viewboxes used to look at the x-ray images each week to allow for optimum viewing conditions. Check the lamps and change bulbs, if needed.
3. Take a phantom image each week to test that the imaging system is functioning properly.

Each week, the mammographer should use an MQSA phantom to take a phantom image. The phantom is a fake breast. The process of taking a phantom image each week helps to check the imaging system's calibrations. The mammographer places the phantom on the image receptor, being careful to align it with the edge of the receptor that is nearest to a patient during a procedure. The mammographer uses both the compression device and the automatic exposure control sensor in the technique specified for a 50% fatty, 50% dense breast compressed to 4.5 centimeters, and takes an image. The mammographer scores, charts, and tracks results of phantom images, so that anomalies in the imaging system are immediately detected and corrected.

Monthly tasks:

1. Visually checks the image system or systems against a written checklist, to ensure nothing is missed
2. Ensures that lights, displays, and mechanical locks are in good working order
3. Tests the rigidity and stability of the equipment

Quarterly tasks:

1. Review records of repeat procedures, analyzing the causes and looking for ways to improve efficiency, reduce costs, and minimize patient exposure
2. Analyze the fixer retention in film to ensure that archived images are stable. How long an image must last varies from state to state, but is a minimum of three years from the date of the procedure, up to 12 years after the patient's last treatment visit. Aim to keep records indefinitely, especially if the patient expresses dissatisfaction with treatment, or threatens a lawsuit, or where the outcome is undesirable, or where the patient was mentally incompetent and then regains competency (e.g., resolved mental illness or operable brain tumor). Keep minors' records until they turn 30.

Semiannual tasks:

1. Darkroom fog analysis to ensure that the darkroom safelights are working properly and that the darkroom is adequately sealed off from exterior light. Unwanted light can fog images as they are developing, reducing the overall quality.
2. Check the film-screen contact. Close contact helps keep image contrast where it needs to be. The cassette is primarily responsible for film-screen contact. The mammographer should clean and test each cassette. If the test film shows dark spots, it may indicate a problem with the film-screen contact. Remove the cassette in question from service until the problem is rectified.
3. Every six months, the mammographer must check that the compression device is in proper working order.

Sources of Motion

There are two kinds of motion that can inhibit the radiographer's ability to take an accurate image: Involuntary and voluntary. Involuntary motions include: Pulses; peristalsis; muscle spasms; shivering due to chills; twitching due to pain; Tourette's syndrome; tics; or Parkinsonian tremors. Voluntary motions come from hostile patients who refuse to be still, patients who are afraid or excited, and attention deficit patients who have difficulty being still. Nervous patients may also unconsciously fidget. Children and elderly patients tend to have a more difficult time being still, as do patients who have chronic pain conditions. If the patient cannot overcome involuntary motions, the radiographer is limited to fast film-speed combinations to offset the effect of the movement.

The radiographer's best tool against voluntary motion is good communication. By communicating what he or she is doing in a clear, polite way that is not condescending, the radiographer can do much to calm nervous, frightened, or hostile patients. While communication is the best tool, the radiographer may need additional strategies in difficult cases. The radiographer can use tape or compression bands to help mobilize body parts. For infants, a Pigg-O-Stat can keep the infant still for the duration of the exposure. Wrapping a child patient in sheets can help the child to stay still and feel secure. The radiographer should take special care to keep the patient comfortable and to answer all questions in straightforward terms that the patient will understand.

Proper Cleaning Procedures

Proper cleaning will help extend the life of the automatic processing unit and will help ensure that it produces accurately developed images. Each day, the radiographer should wash the crossover racks where the film moves from one tank to the next. They should be washed during the start-up and shutdown procedures. The wash tank should also be drained every day. On a weekly basis, the deep racks should be cleaned and the water filters changed. Every month, the processor should be drained entirely and all the tanks and the dryer should be hand cleaned. Fresh developer and fixer solutions should be put in the holding tanks and the developer filter should be changed. At this time, a starter solution should be added to the developer chemicals.

Sensitometric Testing

Periodic sensitometric testing will help to ensure that the automatic processor is working properly and will help the radiographer to recognize any problems early on. The test should be performed on a daily basis. The sensitometric test monitors the processing speed, the image contrast, the developer temperature, and the base plus fog. To perform the test, process a film. During the processing, use a densitometer to measure the speed of the film and the contrast. Match these values with the baseline values for the machine. If they fall within 0.10 units of the baseline, the machine passes the test. The densitometer will also measure an unexposed area of the film for base plus fog, which much not deviate more than 0.05 units from the baseline.

Fluoroscopy

Most radiographic imaging systems are limited to taking a static image of a specific area of the body. In some instances, it is more desirable to view a real-time, fluid image of an internal structure. The static limitation of conventional radiographic techniques is overcome with fluoroscopy. Fluoroscopy allows the radiographer to view the motion of internal structures. During the procedure, it is possible for the radiographer to also capture still shots of specific movements. Many surgical situations call for fluoroscopy, making it a fairly routine procedure, and certainly one with which a radiographer must be familiar. Fluoroscopy uses an x-ray table with the x-ray tube located underneath. The image-detection device is located above the table. (There is some variation in set-up.) During the procedure, the radiologist, radiographer, and surgeon view the live image as it is transferred to a television monitor. Because the patient is exposed for a greater amount of time, fluoroscopy is performed with low milliampere settings, usually around 5mA.

Since the radiographer must view the fluoroscopic image in motion, and because the image may sometimes be dim, the radiographer must know how to compensate. This requires knowledge both of image illumination and of how the eye works. To overcome dim illuminations, the radiographer uses a process called image-intensification. This makes the image much easier to see, and distinguishes different structures within the image better. When viewing a dim object, it helps to know that the eye picks up color in the center of the visual field and views light from around the sides. This means that it is easier to see a dim object by looking at it slightly peripherally. Use peripheral vision when viewing fluoroscopic images.

Cardiovascular and Interventional Technologists

Some of the body's systems are more complex and delicate than others, so the radiographer requires specialized training and procedures for imaging these. For example, imaging vascular structures is a difficult specialty. When a radiographic procedure is used as a treatment, it is referred to as an interventional procedure. Interventional radiologists are physicians who provide radiographic treatment; they require specialized knowledge and additional certification. The most common interventional procedure is angiography, the process of taking an image of an artery. Angiography requires the interventional radiologist or cardiologist to inject a contrast medium into the artery before the imaging takes place. Often, angiography goes hand-in-hand with such procedures as angioplasty, thrombolysis, embolization, vascular stents, and biopsies.

Angiography Procedure

Before:

Patient arrives in Cath Lab after 8-hour fast. Radiologist explains procedure to patient. Patient signs consent forms. Nurse files them.

Nurse infiltrates patient's groin with local anesthetic and shaves site.

Doctor palpates femoral artery in thigh and cleans site with poviodine.

During:

Doctor punctures femoral artery with long (56 mm), large bore, hollow needle (18 or 19 gauge cannula) at 10° angle, which holds artery open. Doctor threads guidewire carefully into femoral artery before removing needle. Doctor moves catheter, attached to end of guidewire, through artery and into needed position.

Doctor injects contrast media into artery to enhance viewing of plaques, aneurysms, etc. Patient feels traveling warmth. Radiographer takes views from several angles. Doctor may insert stent, balloon, etc., based on images. Team monitors for adverse reactions.

After:

Doctor applies pressure and Angioseal to wound. Team monitors patient for: Allergic reaction to contrast media; bleeding and hematoma at entry site; heart attack; stroke; femoral nerve damage; kidney problems. Patient remains still for several hours to avoid complications. Nurse gives heparin per order to prevent blood clot formation.

CT

CT was invented in the early 1930's and became commercially available in 1971. The computed tomographic scanner (CT) works unlike any other imaging system because it does not have a traditional image receptor. As the x-ray beam leaves the patient, the CT scanner measures it with a sophisticated detector, which transmits the data it gathers to a computer. The images the CT captures are 2-D, around a single axis of rotation, but the computer then uses complex mathematical applications to interpret the data and construct a 3-D diagnostic image from it. CT scanners use a very complex series of systems, called windowing, to capture images of higher contrast and detail than would be possible through conventional means. CT eliminates superimposed images out of the field of interest. Toshiba, GE, and Philips manufacture CT scanners with very refined images, up to 256 slices. CT is also called EMI scan, computed axial tomography, CAT scan, and body section roentgenography. CT is losing popularity to MRI, because CT is still expensive.

Contrast Media

While bones absorb x-ray radiation, most soft tissues are penetrated by the radiation, so the contrast between different soft tissue structures is quite low. Soft tissues may be invisible with traditional radiography. If the purpose of the x-ray is to provide diagnostic information about specific soft tissues, such as the gastrointestinal tract, the radiographer must use a contrast media in order to make the area of interest show up better on the film. A contrast media is a substance that absorbs x-rays. For example, if the GI tract needs to be x-rayed, the radiologist may administer a barium sulfate enema prior to the procedure. The barium sulfate will increase the contrast of the gastrointestinal tract, making it easier to distinguish any existing pathologies.

Iodine contrast media often contains royal Tyrian purple dye from marine snails' mucous (Plicopurpura pansa, and Thais kiosquiformis). Patients allergic to shellfish do not necessarily react to iodine contrast media. Ask your patient if he or she has any allergies, and if so, avoid the iodine media, if possible. If you must use iodine media:

- Give corticosteroids before injection, e.g., 32 mg of oral methylprednisolone 12 hours and 2 hours before injecting contrast OR
- Alternatively, give 50 mg of prednisone 13 hours, 7 hours, and one hour prior to contrast injection; add 50 mg of diphenhydramine (decongestant) to the last dose
- Use low-osmolality nonionic agents (3% of patients will still react to these safer but more expensive agents)
- Have the crash cart standing by

Patients with asthma, hyperthyroidism, central myasthenia gravis, sickle cell anemia, allergies, pheochromocytomas, and cardiac arrhythmias are most likely to react; make an allergy alert in these patients' hospital charts.

How to Overcome Test Anxiety

Just the thought of taking a test is enough to make most people a little nervous. A test is an important event that can have a long-term impact on your future, so it's important to take it seriously and it's natural to feel anxious about performing well. But just because anxiety is normal, that doesn't mean that it's helpful in test taking, or that you should simply accept it as part of your life. Anxiety can have a variety of effects. These effects can be mild, like making you feel slightly nervous, or severe, like blocking your ability to focus or remember even a simple detail.

If you experience test anxiety—whether severe or mild—it's important to know how to beat it. To discover this, first you need to understand what causes test anxiety.

Causes of Test Anxiety

While we often think of anxiety as an uncontrollable emotional state, it can actually be caused by simple, practical things. One of the most common causes of test anxiety is that a person does not feel adequately prepared for their test. This feeling can be the result of many different issues such as poor study habits or lack of organization, but the most common culprit is time management. Starting to study too late, failing to organize your study time to cover all of the material, or being distracted while you study will mean that you're not well prepared for the test. This may lead to cramming the night before, which will cause you to be physically and mentally exhausted for the test. Poor time management also contributes to feelings of stress, fear, and hopelessness as you realize you are not well prepared but don't know what to do about it.

Other times, test anxiety is not related to your preparation for the test but comes from unresolved fear. This may be a past failure on a test, or poor performance on tests in general. It may come from comparing yourself to others who seem to be performing better or from the stress of living up to expectations. Anxiety may be driven by fears of the future—how failure on this test would affect your educational and career goals. These fears are often completely irrational, but they can still negatively impact your test performance.

Elements of Test Anxiety

As mentioned earlier, test anxiety is considered to be an emotional state, but it has physical and mental components as well. Sometimes you may not even realize that you are suffering from test anxiety until you notice the physical symptoms. These can include trembling hands, rapid heartbeat, sweating, nausea, and tense muscles. Extreme anxiety may lead to fainting or vomiting. Obviously, any of these symptoms can have a negative impact on testing. It is important to recognize them as soon as they begin to occur so that you can address the problem before it damages your performance.

The mental components of test anxiety include trouble focusing and inability to remember learned information. During a test, your mind is on high alert, which can help you recall information and stay focused for an extended period of time. However, anxiety interferes with your mind's natural processes, causing you to blank out, even on the questions you know well. The strain of testing during anxiety makes it difficult to stay focused, especially on a test that may take several hours. Extreme anxiety can take a huge mental toll, making it difficult not only to recall test information but even to understand the test questions or pull your thoughts together.

Effects of Test Anxiety

Test anxiety is like a disease—if left untreated, it will get progressively worse. Anxiety leads to poor performance, and this reinforces the feelings of fear and failure, which in turn lead to poor performances on subsequent tests. It can grow from a mild nervousness to a crippling condition. If allowed to progress, test anxiety can have a big impact on your schooling, and consequently on your future.

Test anxiety can spread to other parts of your life. Anxiety on tests can become anxiety in any stressful situation, and blanking on a test can turn into panicking in a job situation. But fortunately, you don't have to let anxiety rule your testing and determine your grades. There are a number of relatively simple steps you can take to move past anxiety and function normally on a test and in the rest of life.

Physical Steps for Beating Test Anxiety

While test anxiety is a serious problem, the good news is that it can be overcome. It doesn't have to control your ability to think and remember information. While it may take time, you can begin taking steps today to beat anxiety.

Just as your first hint that you may be struggling with anxiety comes from the physical symptoms, the first step to treating it is also physical. Rest is crucial for having a clear, strong mind. If you are tired, it is much easier to give in to anxiety. But if you establish good sleep habits, your body and mind will be ready to perform optimally, without the strain of exhaustion. Additionally, sleeping well helps you to retain information better, so you're more likely to recall the answers when you see the test questions.

Getting good sleep means more than going to bed on time. It's important to allow your brain time to relax. Take study breaks from time to time so it doesn't get overworked, and don't study right before bed. Take time to rest your mind before trying to rest your body, or you may find it difficult to fall asleep.

Along with sleep, other aspects of physical health are important in preparing for a test. Good nutrition is vital for good brain function. Sugary foods and drinks may give a burst of energy but this burst is followed by a crash, both physically and emotionally. Instead, fuel your body with protein and vitamin-rich foods.

Also, drink plenty of water. Dehydration can lead to headaches and exhaustion, especially if your brain is already under stress from the rigors of the test. Particularly if your test is a long one, drink water during the breaks. And if possible, take an energy-boosting snack to eat between sections.

Along with sleep and diet, a third important part of physical health is exercise. Maintaining a steady workout schedule is helpful, but even taking 5-minute study breaks to walk can help get your blood pumping faster and clear your head. Exercise also releases endorphins, which contribute to a positive feeling and can help combat test anxiety.

When you nurture your physical health, you are also contributing to your mental health. If your body is healthy, your mind is much more likely to be healthy as well. So take time to rest, nourish your body with healthy food and water, and get moving as much as possible. Taking these physical steps will make you stronger and more able to take the mental steps necessary to overcome test anxiety.

Mental Steps for Beating Test Anxiety

Working on the mental side of test anxiety can be more challenging, but as with the physical side, there are clear steps you can take to overcome it. As mentioned earlier, test anxiety often stems from lack of preparation, so the obvious solution is to prepare for the test. Effective studying may be the most important weapon you have for beating test anxiety, but you can and should employ several other mental tools to combat fear.

First, boost your confidence by reminding yourself of past success—tests or projects that you aced. If you're putting as much effort into preparing for this test as you did for those, there's no reason you should expect to fail here. Work hard to prepare; then trust your preparation.

Second, surround yourself with encouraging people. It can be helpful to find a study group, but be sure that the people you're around will encourage a positive attitude. If you spend time with others who are anxious or cynical, this will only contribute to your own anxiety. Look for others who are motivated to study hard from a desire to succeed, not from a fear of failure.

Third, reward yourself. A test is physically and mentally tiring, even without anxiety, and it can be helpful to have something to look forward to. Plan an activity following the test, regardless of the outcome, such as going to a movie or getting ice cream.

When you are taking the test, if you find yourself beginning to feel anxious, remind yourself that you know the material. Visualize successfully completing the test. Then take a few deep, relaxing breaths and return to it. Work through the questions carefully but with confidence, knowing that you are capable of succeeding.

Developing a healthy mental approach to test taking will also aid in other areas of life. Test anxiety affects more than just the actual test—it can be damaging to your mental health and even contribute to depression. It's important to beat test anxiety before it becomes a problem for more than testing.

Study Strategy

Being prepared for the test is necessary to combat anxiety, but what does being prepared look like? You may study for hours on end and still not feel prepared. What you need is a strategy for test prep. The next few pages outline our recommended steps to help you plan out and conquer the challenge of preparation.

STEP 1: SCOPE OUT THE TEST

Learn everything you can about the format (multiple choice, essay, etc.) and what will be on the test. Gather any study materials, course outlines, or sample exams that may be available. Not only will this help you to prepare, but knowing what to expect can help to alleviate test anxiety.

STEP 2: MAP OUT THE MATERIAL

Look through the textbook or study guide and make note of how many chapters or sections it has. Then divide these over the time you have. For example, if a book has 15 chapters and you have five days to study, you need to cover three chapters each day. Even better, if you have the time, leave an extra day at the end for overall review after you have gone through the material in depth.

If time is limited, you may need to prioritize the material. Look through it and make note of which sections you think you already have a good grasp on, and which need review. While you are studying, skim quickly through the familiar sections and take more time on the challenging parts. Write out your plan so you don't get lost as you go. Having a written plan also helps you feel more in control of the study, so anxiety is less likely to arise from feeling overwhelmed at the amount to cover.

STEP 3: GATHER YOUR TOOLS

Decide what study method works best for you. Do you prefer to highlight in the book as you study and then go back over the highlighted portions? Or do you type out notes of the important information? Or is it helpful to make flashcards that you can carry with you? Assemble the pens, index cards, highlighters, post-it notes, and any other materials you may need so you won't be distracted by getting up to find things while you study.

If you're having a hard time retaining the information or organizing your notes, experiment with different methods. For example, try color-coding by subject with colored pens, highlighters, or post-it notes. If you learn better by hearing, try recording yourself reading your notes so you can listen while in the car, working out, or simply sitting at your desk. Ask a friend to quiz you from your flashcards, or try teaching someone the material to solidify it in your mind.

Step 4: Create Your Environment

It's important to avoid distractions while you study. This includes both the obvious distractions like visitors and the subtle distractions like an uncomfortable chair (or a too-comfortable couch that makes you want to fall asleep). Set up the best study environment possible: good lighting and a comfortable work area. If background music helps you focus, you may want to turn it on, but otherwise keep the room quiet. If you are using a computer to take notes, be sure you don't have any other windows open, especially applications like social media, games, or anything else that could distract you. Silence your phone and turn off notifications. Be sure to keep water close by so you stay hydrated while you study (but avoid unhealthy drinks and snacks).

Also, take into account the best time of day to study. Are you freshest first thing in the morning? Try to set aside some time then to work through the material. Is your mind clearer in the afternoon or evening? Schedule your study session then. Another method is to study at the same time of day that you will take the test, so that your brain gets used to working on the material at that time and will be ready to focus at test time.

Step 5: Study!

Once you have done all the study preparation, it's time to settle into the actual studying. Sit down, take a few moments to settle your mind so you can focus, and begin to follow your study plan. Don't give in to distractions or let yourself procrastinate. This is your time to prepare so you'll be ready to fearlessly approach the test. Make the most of the time and stay focused.

Of course, you don't want to burn out. If you study too long you may find that you're not retaining the information very well. Take regular study breaks. For example, taking five minutes out of every hour to walk briskly, breathing deeply and swinging your arms, can help your mind stay fresh.

As you get to the end of each chapter or section, it's a good idea to do a quick review. Remind yourself of what you learned and work on any difficult parts. When you feel that you've mastered the material, move on to the next part. At the end of your study session, briefly skim through your notes again.

But while review is helpful, cramming last minute is NOT. If at all possible, work ahead so that you won't need to fit all your study into the last day. Cramming overloads your brain with more information than it can process and retain, and your tired mind may struggle to recall even previously learned information when it is overwhelmed with last-minute study. Also, the urgent nature of cramming and the stress placed on your brain contribute to anxiety. You'll be more likely to go to the test feeling unprepared and having trouble thinking clearly.

So don't cram, and don't stay up late before the test, even just to review your notes at a leisurely pace. Your brain needs rest more than it needs to go over the information again. In fact, plan to finish your studies by noon or early afternoon the day before the test. Give your brain the rest of the day to relax or focus on other things, and get a good night's sleep. Then you will be fresh for the test and better able to recall what you've studied.

Step 6: Take a Practice Test

Many courses offer sample tests, either online or in the study materials. This is an excellent resource to check whether you have mastered the material, as well as to prepare for the test format and environment.

Check the test format ahead of time: the number of questions, the type (multiple choice, free response, etc.), and the time limit. Then create a plan for working through them. For example, if you have 30 minutes to take a 60-question test, your limit is 30 seconds per question. Spend less time on the questions you know well so that you can take more time on the difficult ones.

If you have time to take several practice tests, take the first one open book, with no time limit. Work through the questions at your own pace and make sure you fully understand them. Gradually work up to taking a test under test conditions: sit at a desk with all study materials put away and set a timer. Pace yourself to make sure you finish the test with time to spare and go back to check your answers if you have time.

After each test, check your answers. On the questions you missed, be sure you understand why you missed them. Did you misread the question (tests can use tricky wording)? Did you forget the information? Or was it something you hadn't learned? Go back and study any shaky areas that the practice tests reveal.

Taking these tests not only helps with your grade, but also aids in combating test anxiety. If you're already used to the test conditions, you're less likely to worry about it, and working through tests until you're scoring well gives you a confidence boost. Go through the practice tests until you feel comfortable, and then you can go into the test knowing that you're ready for it.

Test Tips

On test day, you should be confident, knowing that you've prepared well and are ready to answer the questions. But aside from preparation, there are several test day strategies you can employ to maximize your performance.

First, as stated before, get a good night's sleep the night before the test (and for several nights before that, if possible). Go into the test with a fresh, alert mind rather than staying up late to study.

Try not to change too much about your normal routine on the day of the test. It's important to eat a nutritious breakfast, but if you normally don't eat breakfast at all, consider eating just a protein bar. If you're a coffee drinker, go ahead and have your normal coffee. Just make sure you time it so that the caffeine doesn't wear off right in the middle of your test. Avoid sugary beverages, and drink enough water to stay hydrated but not so much that you need a restroom break 10 minutes into the test. If your test isn't first thing in the morning, consider going for a walk or doing a light workout before the test to get your blood flowing.

Allow yourself enough time to get ready, and leave for the test with plenty of time to spare so you won't have the anxiety of scrambling to arrive in time. Another reason to be early is to select a good seat. It's helpful to sit away from doors and windows, which can be distracting. Find a good seat, get out your supplies, and settle your mind before the test begins.

When the test begins, start by going over the instructions carefully, even if you already know what to expect. Make sure you avoid any careless mistakes by following the directions.

Then begin working through the questions, pacing yourself as you've practiced. If you're not sure on an answer, don't spend too much time on it, and don't let it shake your confidence. Either skip it and come back later, or eliminate as many wrong answers as possible and guess among the remaining ones. Don't dwell on these questions as you continue—put them out of your mind and focus on what lies ahead.

Be sure to read all of the answer choices, even if you're sure the first one is the right answer. Sometimes you'll find a better one if you keep reading. But don't second-guess yourself if you do immediately know the answer. Your gut instinct is usually right. Don't let test anxiety rob you of the information you know.

If you have time at the end of the test (and if the test format allows), go back and review your answers. Be cautious about changing any, since your first instinct tends to be correct, but make sure you didn't misread any of the questions or accidentally mark the wrong answer choice. Look over any you skipped and make an educated guess.

At the end, leave the test feeling confident. You've done your best, so don't waste time worrying about your performance or wishing you could change anything. Instead, celebrate the successful completion of this test. And finally, use this test to learn how to deal with anxiety even better next time.

Review Video: Test Anxiety
Visit mometrix.com/academy and enter code: 100340

Important Qualification

Not all anxiety is created equal. If your test anxiety is causing major issues in your life beyond the classroom or testing center, or if you are experiencing troubling physical symptoms related to your anxiety, it may be a sign of a serious physiological or psychological condition. If this sounds like your situation, we strongly encourage you to seek professional help.

Online Resources

Due to our efforts to try to keep this book to a manageable length, we've created a link that will give you access to all of your online resources:

mometrix.com/resources719/cres

It's Your Moment, Let's Celebrate It!

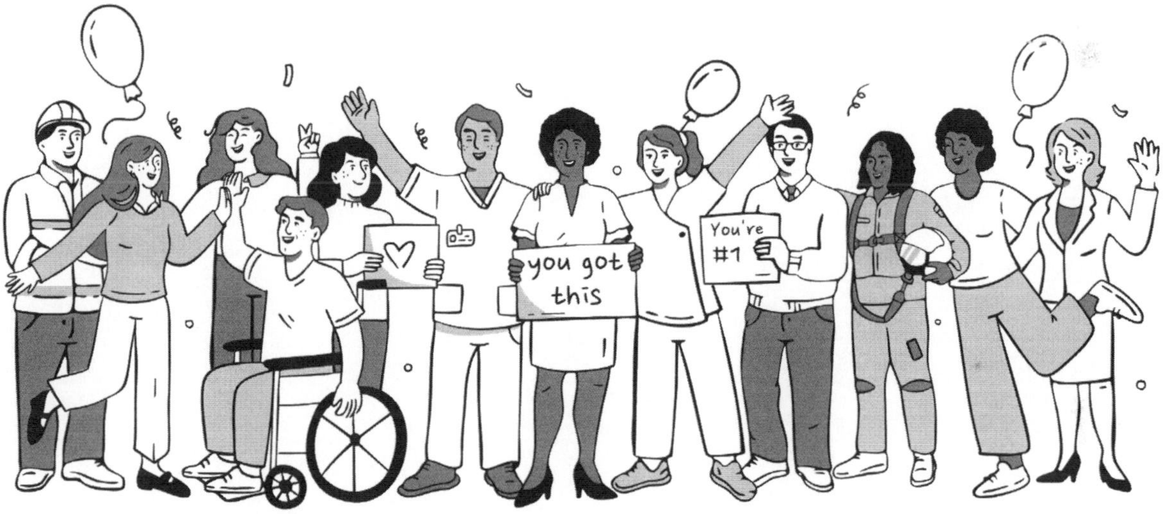

Share your story @mometrixtestpreparation